MRI of the Brain II:
Non-Neoplastic Disease

The Raven MRI Teaching File

Series Editors

Robert B. Lufkin
William G. Bradley, Jr.
Michael Brant-Zawadzki

MRI of the Brain II: Non-Neoplastic Disease

Editors

Michael Brant-Zawadzki, M.D., F.A.C.R.
Director of MRI
Hoag Memorial Hospital
Newport Beach, California

William G. Bradley, Jr., M.D., Ph.D.
Director of MRI and Radiology Research
Long Beach Memorial Medical Center
Long Beach, California

Raven Press New York

Raven Press, 1185 Avenue of the Americas, New York, New York 10036

Made in the United States of America

Library of Congress Cataloging-in-Publication Data

MRI of the brain: non-neoplastic disease/editors, William G.
   Bradley, Jr., Michael Brant-Zawadzki.
      p. cm.—(The Raven MRI teaching file)
   Includes bibliographical references and index.
   ISBN 0-88167-745-0 (v. 1).—ISBN 0-88167-696-9 (v. 2)
   1. Brain—Magnetic resonance imaging. I. Bradley, William G.
II. Brant-Zawadzki, Michael. III. Series.
   [DNLM: 1. Brain Diseases—diagnosis. 2. Magnetic Resonance
Imaging. WL 348 M939]
RC386.6.M34M76 1989
616.8'047548—dc20
DNLM/DLC
for Library of Congress

            90-9107
            CIP

9 8 7 6 5 4 3 2 1

To all the residents and fellows in Radiology and Neuroradiology who gave their time and efforts to help us in our many tasks recently and in the past.

Magnetic Resonance Imaging (MRI) is a complex, rapidly evolving modality which has recently developed applications in all areas of diagnostic radiology. The successful radiologist in the 1990s *must* be proficient at MRI. To develop such proficiency is a formidable task, particularly for radiologists who were not exposed to MRI during their residencies. This 1,000 case MR teaching file is intended to help the practicing radiologist rapidly acquire a storehouse of experience which should aid development of proficiency in MRI. Cases have been carefully selected to show variable manifestations of common pathology as well as the occasional unusual case. The discussions have been kept brief, conforming to the teaching file format. If the reader focuses first on the left hand page while covering the right hand page, retention of information is significantly improved. Although the diagnosis in these workbooks is often suggested by the clinical history and presentation of selected images, the same information of the entire series is available in a convenient single video disk in which the reader is given the option to either choose the selected images reproduced in the printed workbooks or additional images including color and "movie" sequences from the complete imaging file. Additionally, the video disk format allows case presentation either with or without clinical information or orientation to a particular organ system. The video disk is available through Medical Interactive, 3708 Mt. Diablo Boulevard, Suite 120, Lafayette, California 94549.

The series editors would like to thank the section editors for their efforts in organizing the individual 100 case workbooks. This represents contributions from a large number of our friends and colleagues. This also allows us to show cases from a wide variety of manufacturers, MR instruments using a range of magnetic field strengths. We would also like to thank Mary Rogers and her staff at Raven Press for all their help and encouragement during the course of this project.

Robert B. Lufkin, M.D.
William G. Bradley, Jr., M.D., Ph.D.
Michael Brant-Zawadzki, M.D., F.A.C.R.

Volumes I and II of the Raven MRI Teaching File focus on nonneoplastic diseases of the brain. Volume I focuses on flow phenomena, vascular abnormalities, hemorrhage, and trauma, while Volume II focuses on hydrocephalus, infarction, and demyelinating disease. Although these topics are emphasized and thus provide some differentiation of Volumes I and II, in general, they should be taken together as there is considerable overlap.

The cases in these volumes are arranged in order and should be approached in sequence. The reader will get the most out of each case if the key images and history are reviewed on the left hand page prior to reading the diagnosis and discussion on the right hand page.

Michael Brant-Zawadzki, M.D., F.A.C.R.
William G. Bradley, Jr., M.D., Ph.D.

Acknowledgments

Cases in both volumes have come from high field and mid field systems at Hoag and Huntington, as well as from the systems of many of our colleagues who have either sent us interesting cases or asked us for a second opinion. We thank them for allowing us to use their cases in this teaching file series. We also thank those who have been indispensable in putting this teaching file together. At Huntington these were the 1989–1990 MR Fellows, Stephen Davis, M.D. and Louis Teresi, M.D.; technologists, Leslee Watson, Jose Jimenez, Laurel Adler, and Sheri Gregory. We thank Denise Longpre for manuscript preparation and Kaye Finley for everything else.

At Hoag, we thank, in particular, Janet Arnds for manuscript preparation, Jim Walling, Debbie Norman, Susan Steward, Jackie Oldeck, Kevin O'Brien who helped in case procurement and aides Arik Killion and Micah Eaton who helped with case selection. Without their efforts, this task would have been much more onerous.

MRI of the Brain II:
Non-Neoplastic Disease

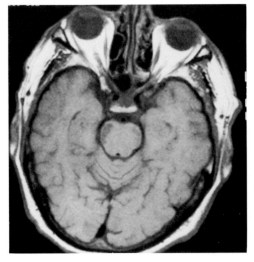

FIG. 1A. SE 650/20.

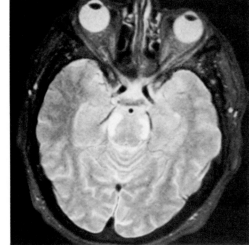

FIG. 1B. SE 2,800/70.

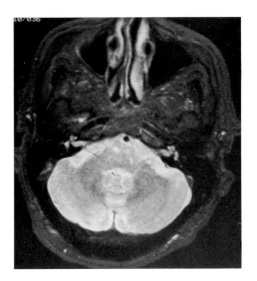

FIG. 1C. SE 2,800/70.

Clinical History

A 61-year-old male with progressive gait disorder, limb weakness and dysarthria.

Findings

The T1-weighted axial sequence at the level of the pons (1A) shows a curvilinear area of low signal intensity along the right pontine periphery corresponding to the cortical spinal tract. A similar, less discernible focus of low intensity is seen on the left-hand side.

The T2-weighted axial sequence shows elevation of signal intensity in the region of the pontine cortical spinal tracts, extending down to the pyramids in the medulla (1B, 1C).

Diagnosis

Amyotrophic lateral sclerosis (ALS).

Discussion

ALS is a disease of middle and late life that is familial and presumably inherited in 8–10% of the cases. The pathology is not specific but highly stylized anatomically with the large motor neurons of the anterior horn cells showing marked reduction in numbers. Consequently, anterior roots become atrophic. Brain-stem motor nuclei are also afflicted. Degeneration of the cortical spinal tracts accompanies this and is nonspecific with the demyelination presumably secondary in nature. Although more protracted cases can be seen, death usually occurs within five years of onset due to respiratory and/or oropharyngeal compromise.

The magnetic resonance (MR) scan nicely delineates the involvement of the cortical spinal tracts in this particular patient. The clinical history, the bilaterality of the disorder as shown on MR is helpful at arriving at the clinical diagnosis.

Reference

1. Munsat TL. Adult motor neuron diseases. In: *Merritt's textbook of neurology.* Philadelphia: Lea and Feberger, 1989;683–685.

Submitted by: Walter Kucharczyk, M.D., Toronto General Hospital, Toronto, Canada; Michael Brant-Zawadzki, M.D., Senior Editor.

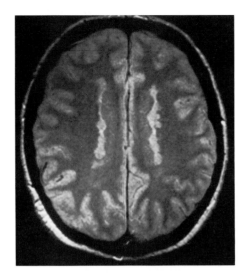

FIG. 2A. SE 2,700/30.

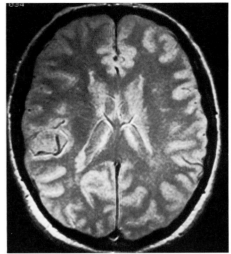

FIG. 2B. SE 2,700/30.

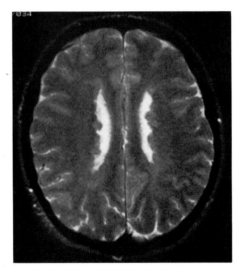

FIG. 2C. SE 2,700/80.

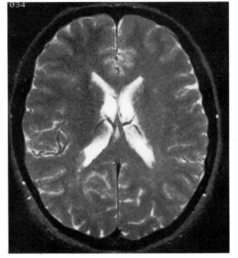

FIG. 2D. SE 2,700/80.

Clinical History

A 38-year-old female with seizures.

Findings

The first (2A, 2B) and second echo images (2C, 2D) show a multi-lobulated appearance to the outer lateral ventricular walls. This is due to multiple foci of isointense signal in a nodular distribution along the subependymal region.

Diagnosis

Typical gray matter heterotopia.

Discussion

The migrational disorder represented by gray matter heterotopia is generally diagnosed in childhood due to intractable seizures. However, it may go unrecognized until adulthood and be presumed due to idiopathic epilepsy if no imaging studies are done. The most typical form of heterotopia is the one shown in this particular case. The differential diagnosis could include tuberous sclerosis, but in that entity the lesions are generally of higher signal intensity on T2-weighted images, are associated with subcortical tubers of a larger size, and also the classic facial features. Calcification is also seen in tuberous sclerosis but absent in gray matter heterotopia. Other tumors, such as metastatic ones, would also have altered signal intensity.

References

1. Vanderknaap MS, Valk J. Classification of congenital abnormalities of the CNS. *AJNR* 1988;9:315–326.
2. Barkovich AJ, Chuang SH, Norman D. MR of neuronal migration anomalies. *AJNR* 1987;8:1009–1017.

Submitted by: Michael Brant-Zawadzki, M.D., Senior Editor.

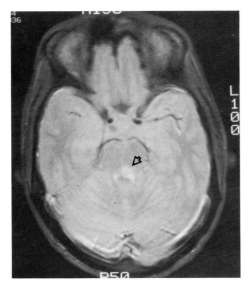

FIG. 3A. SE 2,800/35.

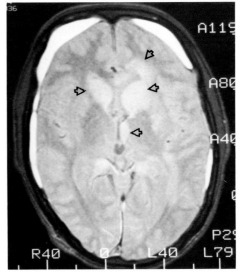

FIG. 3B. SE 2,800/35.

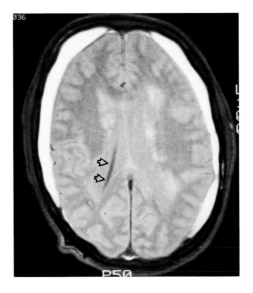

FIG. 3C. SE 2,800/35.

Clinical History

A human immunodeficiency virus (HIV) positive 24-year-old male with altered mental status, status-post ventricular shunting.

Findings

First echo of the T2-weighted axial sequence shows multiple lesions in a subependymal distribution of the ventricular system. Note the high signal intensity focus in the left paramedian pontine tegmentum (3A, arrow) as well as multiple foci along the frontal horn, third ventricle, and lateral-ventricular ependyma (3B). Note also the signal-void linear defect produced by the intraventricular shunt (3C), the subependymal portions of the ventricles again containing multiple high signal foci. Bilateral extra-axial collections of blood are seen in the subdural space.

Diagnosis

1. Cryptococcal meningitis, status post-hydrocephalus and shunting with resulting subdural hematomas.
2. Basal ganglia, subependymal cryptococcal cerebritis.

Discussion

Prior pathologic literature has shown that cryptococcal organisms spread through the perivascular spaces of the arteries perforating the brain from the basal cisterns. Such spread through the Virchow-Robin spaces ultimately propagates the infection into the basal ganglia, internal capsule, thalamus, and brain stem. The changes appear relatively characteristic for cryptococcosis, which generally incites no host response in the form of perifocal edema or enhancement. However, given the multiplicity of afflictions that can occur in immunocompromised patients, absolute specificity is not obtainable with MRI or any other imaging technique.

It has recently been noted that AIDS may have neurologic symptoms as the initial complaint in approximately 10% of all patients. Ultimately, as many as 25% of patients with AIDS will ultimately have focal CT abnormalities.

Other infectious etiologies common in AIDS patients include toxoplasmosis, coccidioidomycosis, cytomegalo virus, and HIV itself. The latter affliction generally presents as a diffuse picture of atrophy with elevation of signal intensity throughout the deep hemispheric white matter in a homogeneous fashion rather than in more local manifestations of infections seen in the other entities.

Incidentally, bilateral subdural hematomas can occur following shunt decompression of the intraventricular system due to the relatively rapid shrinkage of the brain following the ventriculostomy and resultant stretching of the bridging cortical veins and their disruption. For this reason, the shunt placed in a prominently dilated ventricular system is often accompanied by a valve that can control the rate of ventricular fluid decompression.

References

1. Wehn SM, Heinz ER, Burger PC, et al. Dilated Virchow-Robin spaces and cryptococcal meningitis associated with AIDS: CT and MR findings. *J Comp Assist Tomogr* 1989;13:5:756–762.
2. Ramsey RG, Geremia GK. CNS complications of AIDS: CT and MR findings. *AJR* 1988;151:449–454.
3. Jarvik JG, Hesselink J, Kennedy C, et al. Acquired immune deficiency syndrome. Magnetic resonance patterns of brain involvement with pathologic correlation. *Arch Neurol* 1988;45:731–736.

Submitted by: Walter Kucharczyk, M.D., Toronto General Hospital, Toronto, Canada; Michael Brant-Zawadzki, M.D., Senior Editor.

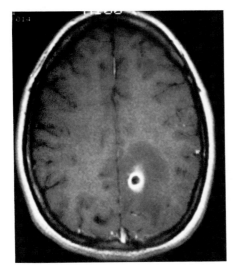

FIG. 4A. SE 600/20 with Gd-DTPA.

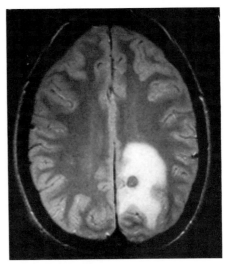

FIG. 4B. SE 2,700/30.

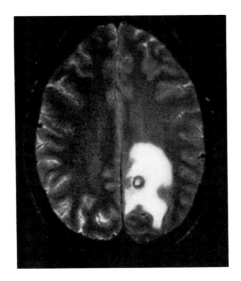

FIG. 4C. SE 2,700/80.

Clinical History

A 37-year-old female with first-time seizure.

Findings

The T1-weighted image obtained after intravenous injection of paramagnetic contrast shows a ring-enhancing lesion in the left paramedian parietal subcortical region with lowered signal intensity of the surrounding white matter. The first and second echo images of the T2-weighted sequence (4B, 4C) verify the prominent vasogenic edema surrounding a small, ring-like lesion with central high signal on the second echo indicating necrotic or liquid center. No other lesions were seen on this scan. The patient was a white, Anglo-Saxon female with no significant travel history except for a brief visit to Tijuana, Mexico several months previously.

Diagnosis

Cysticercosis.

Discussion

The MR appearance here is quite typical for a small abscess. The discrete, ring-like appearance of the lesion with a necrotic core and marked reactive vasogenic edema typify small inflammatory lesions. Occasional metastatic foci and even primary malignant gliomas can show this appearance. The diagnosis of cysticercosis was not suspected given the ethnic background of the patient. The only clue was the recent trip to Mexico.

Occasionally, neuro-cysticercosis may present as a single parenchymal lesion. In such cases, the diagnosis often rests on surgical proof. Given the well-formed capsule, such extirpation of the lesion may be relatively easy. The death of the larva can incite a very dramatic inflammatory response, prior to subsequent calcification of the lesion in the brain. In fact, the calcification may eventually disappear. It may well be that some of the focal infections remain subclinical.

References

1. Zee CS, Segall HD, Miller C, et al. Unusual neuroradiological features of intracranial cysticercosis. *Radiology* 1980;137:397–407.
2. Carbajal JR, Palacios E, Azar-Kia B. Radiology of cysticercosis of the central nervous system including computed tomography. *Radiology* 1977;125:127–131.
3. Cardenas J. Cysticercosis of the nervous system: pathologic and radiologic findings. *J Neurosurg* 1962;19:635–649.
4. Suh DC, Chang KH, Han MH. Unusual MR manifestations of neurocysticercosis. *Neuroradiology* 1989;31:396–402.

Submitted by: Paul Stern, M.D., Glendora Radiology Associates, San Gabriel Valley, California; Michael Brant-Zawadzki, M.D., Senior Editor.

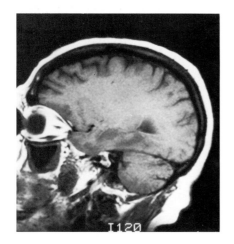

FIG. 5A. SE 600/20.

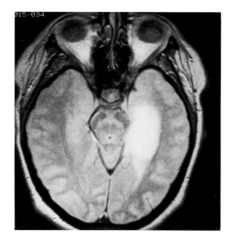

FIG. 5B. SE 2,700/30.

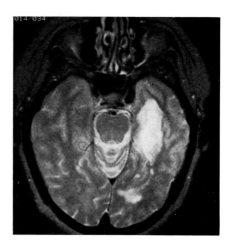

FIG. 5C. SE 2,700/80.

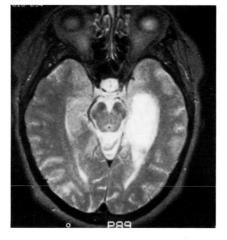

FIG. 5D. SE 2,700/80.

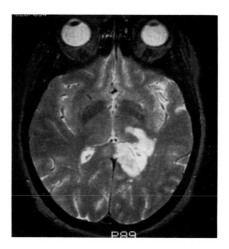

FIG. 5E. SE 2,700/80.

Clinical History

A 56-year-old female with acute mental status change and memory loss.

Findings

The T1-weighted and dual-echo T2-weighted images obtained on admission (5A–5E) show a diffuse abnormality of the deep left temporal lobe, extending from the uncus along the temporal horn to the region of the left atrium, and into the calcar avis of the occipital lobe. The lesion is reasonably well delineated, with mild-mass effect seen. It does appear to spare the basal ganglia except for a small amount of posterior-lateral thalamic involvement. Note that the followup scan obtained three months later (5F, 5G) shows marked diminution of the lesion size, at a time when the patient was clinically normal.

Diagnosis

Herpes encephalitis.

Discussion

Herpes simplex encephalitis is an uncommon, potentially fatal disease, but one that can now be treated with Acyclovir. For optimum outcome, rapid diagnosis and institution of therapy are paramount—this occurred in the patient presented. It has been suggested that MRI may be more sensitive than CT in detecting the early stages of herpes simplex encephalitis. Pathologically, the disease process is characterized by hemorrhagic necrosis involving one or both temporal lobes. Therefore, when bilateral temporal lobe lesions are seen, particularly if foci of hemorrhage are present within, in a patient with acute mental status deterioration, the diagnosis of herpes encephalitis is relatively easy. Nevertheless, in most instances, the patient is treated presumptively in the appropriate clinical setting even with negative imaging studies.

The differential diagnosis includes bilateral temporal lobe infarction and temporal glioma or gliomatosis. The acuteness of symptom onset, and progression of disease generally are strong clues to the presence of herpes encephalitis. However, occasionally angiography may be necessary to help exclude vascular occlusive disease as the etiology for the abnormalities seen.

References

1. Lester JW, Carter NP, Reynolds TL. Herpes encephalitis: MR monitoring of response to Acyclovir therapy. *J Comput Assist Tomogr* 1988;12:941–943.
2. Neils EW, Lukin R, Tomsick T, et al. Magnetic resonance imaging and computed tomography scanning of herpes simplex encephalitis. *J Neurosurg* 1987;67:592–594.
3. Schroth G, Gawehn J, Thron A, et al. Early diagnosis of herpes simplex encephalitis by MRI. *Neurology* 1987;37:179–183.
4. Whitley RJ, Soong SJ, Linneman C, et al. Herpes simplex encephalitis—clinical assessment. *JAMA* 1982;247:317–320.

Submitted by: Paul Stern, M.D., Glendora Radiology Associates, San Gabriel Valley, California; Michael Brant-Zawadzki, M.D., Senior Editor.

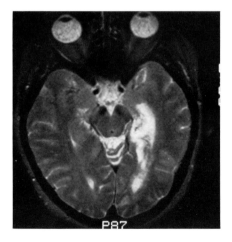 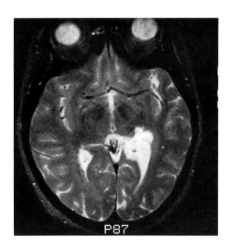

FIG. 5F. SE 2,700/80.   FIG. 5G. SE 2,700/80.

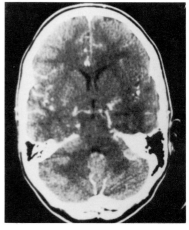
FIG. 6A. CT with contrast.

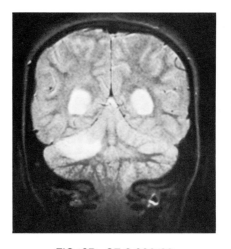
FIG. 6B. SE 2,000/80.

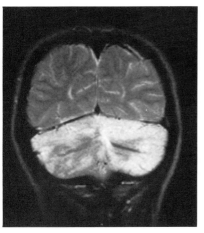
FIG. 6C. SE 2,300/80.

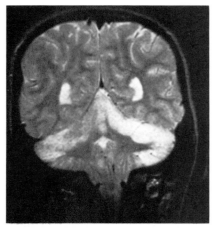
FIG. 6D. SE 2,800/80.

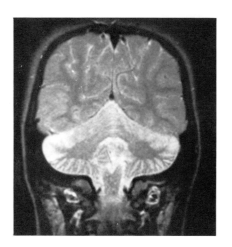
FIG. 6E. SE 2,800/80.

Clinical History

A young female with dizziness, nausea, vomiting, and generalized weakness. Sudden onset of seizure and unusual arm movements prompted CT scan in early March. Two weeks later, patient continued to have cerebellar signs including truncal ataxia and vomiting and an MR exam was done (6B–6D). Illness slowly resolved by July (6E).

Findings

The initial CT scan (6A) shows no definite abnormality in the cerebellum. However, the MR study obtained three days later shows definite abnormality in the right cerebellum consisting of high signal intensity in the right superior cerebellar hemisphere. This progressed over the next ten days (6C) to bilateral cerebellar involvement with diffuse distribution, particularly on the left. By July, when the symptoms of the disease had abated clinically, the MR picture was returning toward normal with only a small region of the superior right cerebellum showing elevated signal intensity. The patient continued on to a full recovery.

Diagnosis

Viral cerebellar-"itis".

Discussion

Only scant literature exists on the MR appearance of encephalitides, particularly those confined to the posterior fossa. Viral encephalitis can manifest diffusely throughout the brain or in a localized fashion (such as herpes encephalitis in the tempora lobe). Cerebellar infection can occur with a nonspecific syndrome such as the one described here. The reason for the localization is unknown. Causes of acute viral encephalitis include enteroviruses, measles, mumps, rubella, chicken pox, as well as the arthropod-borne viruses responsible for epidemic encephalitis.

The MR imaging is nonspecific in this and other cases. The differential diagnosis would include inflammatory, ischemic, demyelinating diseases. The probability of infection is heightened by the progression of disease on the serial studies.

References

1. Hosoda K, Tamaki N, Masumura M, et al. Magnetic resonance images of brain stem encephalitis. *J Neurosurg* 1987;66:283–285.
2. Weiner L, Fleming J. Viral infections of the nervous system. *J Neurosurg* 1984;61:207–224.

Submitted by: Paul Stern, M.D., Glendora Radiology Associates, San Gabriel, California; Michael Brant-Zawadzki, M.D., Senior Editor.

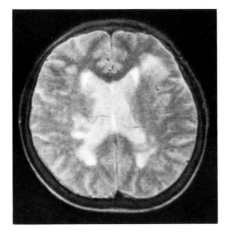 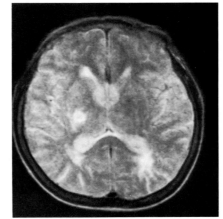

FIG. 7A. SE 2,150/100.   FIG. 7B. SE 2,150/100.

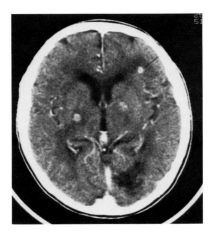

FIG. 7C. CT with contrast.

Clinical History

A 70-year-old female with fever and dehydration.

Findings

Multiple foci of high signal intensity are seen on the T2-weighted images (0.5T) in the white matter, as well as in the region of the right internal capsule. The latter lesion particularly shows a "target" like appearance. The contrast enhanced CT scan confirms the micro abscess-like picture in this case.

Diagnosis

Nocardiosis.

Discussion

Nocardial infection is generally considered unusual and one that occurs in immunocompromised patients. However, no underlying abnormality of the immune system is found in up to 49% of the patients in one series (*see* Palmer et al., ref. 2). The respiratory tract is the usual site of entry, lung involvement being seen in 70% of the reported cases. The central nervous system (CNS) is by far the most common secondary site of infection.

The differential diagnosis on the MRI would include microangiopathic disease of any etiology, as well as any hematogenous infectious process.

The MR findings would be perhaps similar to those seen in elderly patients with micro-angiopathic leukoencephalomalacia were it not for the target-like appearance of the right internal capsule lesion (7A, 7B). The contrast-enhanced CT strongly suggests multiple small abscesses (7C). This case makes the point that intravenous contrast can be quite valuable in differentiating small, deep hemispheric abnormalities even in elderly patients. The MR scan was obtained prior to the availability of intravenous paramagnetic contrast agents.

References

1. Schroth et al. Advantage of magnetic resonance imaging in the diagnosis of cerebral infections. *Neuroradiology* 1987;29:120–126.
2. Palmer D et al. Diagnostic and therapeutic consideration in Nocardia Asteroides infection. *Medicine* 1974;53:391–401.
3. Brant-Zawadzki M et al. NMR imaging of experimental brain abscess: comparison with CT. *AJNR* 1983;4:250–253.
4. Salaki et al. Fungal and yeast infections of the central nervous system: a clinical review. *Medicine* 1984;63:108–132.
5. Sze G. Infections and inflammatory diseases. In: Stark DD, Bradley WG, eds. *Magnetic resonance imaging.* St. Louis: C.V. Mosby Co., 1988;317–343.

Submitted by: Michael Brant-Zawadzki, M.D., Senior Editor.

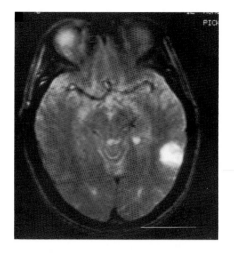

FIG. 8A. SE 2,500/100.

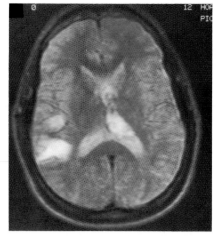

FIG. 8B. SE 2,500/100.

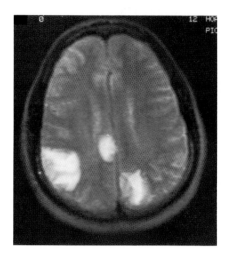

FIG. 8C. SE 2,500/100.

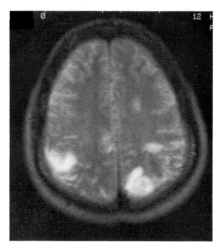

FIG. 8D. SE 2,500/100.

Clinical History

AIDS, altered mental status.

Findings

Multifocal areas of high signal intensity are scattered throughout the subcortical white matter with a lesion in the left thalamus also shown. The lesion in the posterior right paramedian parietal region suggests a target-like appearance (8A–8D).

Diagnosis

Toxoplasmosis.

Discussion

Patients with AIDS are prone to multiple abnormalities involving their brains. Multifocal abscesses due to toxoplasmosis are a common finding in MR scans of these patients. The differentiation from other multifocal disease such as lymphoma may be difficult, even when the target-like nature of the lesions exist. Vasogenic edema sways one toward diagnosing an inflammatory process, although, again, lymphoma can produce a similar picture.

Diffuse white-matter abnormality can be seen due to a primary HIV infection and may be quite subtle. More focal white-matter abnormality can be due to progressive, multi-focal leukoencephalopathy—this entity does not exhibit mass effect, however. In general, when the MR scan shows multi-focal abnormalities, treatment for toxoplasmosis will generally be begun presumptively. A brain biopsy can be done to help guide the management. Occasionally, concurrent infection, lymphoma, Kaposi's sarcoma, and/or progressive multifocal leukoencephalopathy or primary HIV infection can exist. Atrophy is a common accompaniment of the latter entity.

References

1. Zee C et al. MR imaging of cerebral toxoplasmosis: correlation of computed tomography and pathology. *J Comput Assist Tomogr* 1985;9(4):797–799.
2. Jarvik J. Acquired immunodeficiency syndrome: magnetic resonance patterns of brain involvement with pathologic correlation. *Arch Neurol* 1988;45:731–736.
3. Ramsey R. CNS complications of AIDS: CT and MR findings. *AJR* 1988;151:449–454.

Submitted by: Michael Brant-Zawadzki, M.D., Senior Editor.

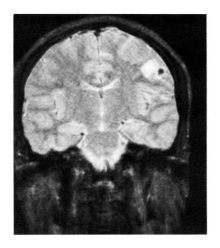 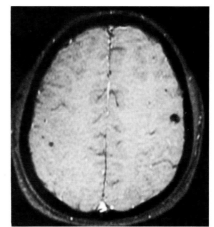

FIG. 9A. SE 2,800/70.   FIG. 9B. GRE 250/15/50°.

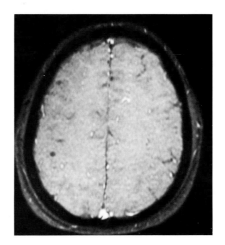

FIG. 9C. GRE 250/15/50°.

Clinical History

Seizures; young Mexican male.

Findings

The T2-weighted image (9A) shows a punctate area of low signal intensity surrounded by high signal in the white matter that is typical for vasogenic edema. This was the only lesion seen on the routine MR sequences. The GRASS (gradient echo) sequence (9B, 9C) shows several other small punctate foci of low signal intensity scattered throughout the brain parenchyma in a subcortical location.

Diagnosis

Cysticercosis.

Discussion

Cysticercosis (pork tapeworm) is the most common cause of seizures in Mexico. Parenchymal cysticercosis of the brain results when the larva is carried to the brain through the hematogenous route. An inflammatory response ensues. The larva then dies and calcifies. Thus parenchymal cysticercosis may show in several stages within the brain. The inflammatory stage is nonspecific, generally in the subcortical region, and may simulate a neoplasm or other infection. With calcification of the larva, the diagnosis becomes more obvious. The late stage shows only punctate calcification. Eventually, this may fade. The gradient echo sequences are more sensitive to small foci of calcification due to the magnetic susceptibility difference between the normal brain and calcium. Therefore, such sequences can be a useful adjunct for detection of punctate foci of calcium.

Brain cysticercosis may have two other presentations beyond the parenchymal one. Racemose, or meningeal cysticercosis can occur due to a larval infection of the meninges with cyst formation there. This has the clinical presentation of a chronic meningitis. Also, ventricular cysticercosis can occur with cysts producing obstructive hydrocephalus within any portion of the ventricular system.

References

1. Zee C et al. MR imaging of neurocysticercosis. *J Comput Assist Tomogr* 1988;12(6):927–934.
2. Rhee R. MR imaging of intraventricular cysticercosis. *J Comput Assist Tomogr* 1987;11(4):598–601.
3. Suss R et al. MR imaging of intracranial cysticercosis: comparison with CT and anatomopathologic features. *AJNR* 1986;7:235–242.

Submitted by: Michael Brant-Zawadzki, M.D., Senior Editor.

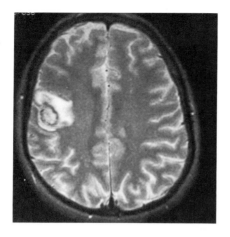
FIG. 10A. May 19, 1988, SE 2,800/70.

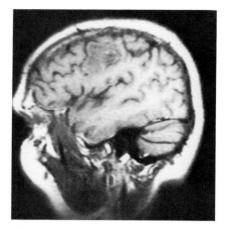
FIG. 10B. May 19, 1988, SE 600/20.

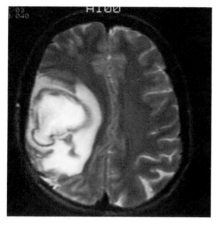
FIG. 10C. May 26, 1988, SE 2,800/70.

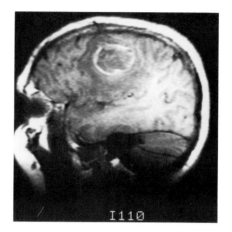
FIG. 10D. May 26, 1988, SE 600/20.

Clinical History

Three episodes of left facial, arm, and leg numbness and possible weakness with resolution prompted the initial MRI study. Progressive weakness and mental status change occurred.

Findings

The initial study (May 19) shows a focal area of white matter high signal in the subcortical right parietal cortex on the T2-weighted sequence (10A) within which lies a garland-shaped lesion, the border of which shows low signal intensity. Mild-mass effect is present. The sagittal T1-weighted sequence shows low signal within the affected area (10B). The scans of May 26, obtained one week later, show marked progression of the abnormality with much greater vasogenic edema, the lesion itself extending from the subcortical region to the periventricular white matter, as shown on the T2-weighted axial image (10C). The border of the lesion now contains high signal intensity and is still somewhat irregular on the T1-weighted sagittal sequence (10D).

Diagnosis

Brain abscess.

Discussion

This appearance is quite typical for the evolution of a cerebritis into an early abscess of the brain. The typical early cerebritis picture is nonspecific with subcortical location of edema being first seen (due to the hematogenous route of spread into the capillary system). The presence of a low signal border on the T2-weighted images signifies an early attempt at capsule formation and collagen deposition around the infected site. The subsequent progression to a larger border with hemorrhagic components is typical for the development of the micro-hemorrhages within the early-abscessed capsule. A successful host response would proceed to form a thick, regular ring surrounding the abscess (see next case). However, inadequate or delayed treatment will produce progressive spread of the cerebritis with the medial wall particularly prone to involvement due to difficulty in obtaining vascular ingrowth from the periphery of the brain to the deeper portions of the abscessed capsule. Although the initial MR appearance of the lesion is non-specific, the very rapid progression strongly suggests an inflammatory etiology. Further questioning revealed that dental work several weeks before led to gum inflammation in this patient, presumably the source of infection.

References

1. Schroth M et al. Advantage of magnetic resonance imaging in the diagnosis of cerebral infections. *Neuroradiology* 1987;29:120–126.
2. Brant-Zawadzki M et al. NMR imaging of experimental brain abscess: comparison with CT. *AJNR* 4:250–253.
3. Salaki M et al. Fungal and yeast infections of the central nervous system: a clinical review. *Medicine* 1984;63:108–132.
4. Sze G. Infections and inflammatory diseases. In: Stark DD, Bradley WG, eds. *Magnetic resonance imaging.* St. Louis: C.V. Mosby Co., 1988;317–343.
5. Rosenbloom M et al. Decreased mortality from brain abscess since advent of computerized tomography. *J Neurosurg* 1978;49:658–668.
6. Enzman D et al. Experimental brain abscess evolution: computed tomographic and neuropathologic correlation. *Radiology* 1979;133:113–122.

Submitted by: Michael Brant-Zawadzki, M.D., Senior Editor.

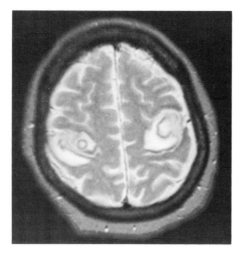

FIG. 11A. October 16, 1989, SE 2,800/80.

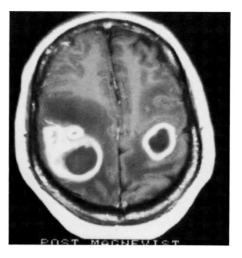

FIG. 11B. October 16, 1989, SE 5,000/20 with Gd-DTPA.

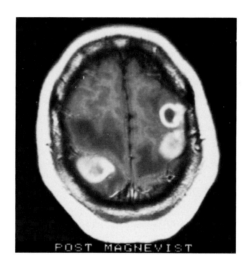

FIG. 11C. October 16, 1989, SE 5,000/20 with Gd-DTPA.

Clinical History

A 61-year-old female with urinary tract infection, headaches.

Findings

The first study, done on September 15, 1989, shows an appearance of the two lesions of the high parietal convexities quite similar to that described in the prior case. Ring- and garland-shaped lesions, the borders of which are low in signal intensity, are surrounded by high signal in the surrounding white matter with mild-mass effect (11A). At this time, the abnormalities were attributed to ischemia, and the patient was placed on antibiotics for her co-existent urinary tract infection.

One month later, the patient's mental status had deteriorated, prompting hospitalization. A repeat study was done with paramagnetic contrast injection. This study documents the progression of the lesions into larger, ring-shaped entities. The right-sided lesion shows a daughter budding lesion off the anterior capsule (11B, 11C).

Diagnosis

Brain abscess—*Staphylococcus aureus.*

Discussion

This case demonstrates the progression of partially treated cerebritis into a well-encapsulated abscess. The antibiotics used for the urinary tract infection were inadequate for treating this brain abscess, accounting for the subacute but progressive course. The appearance of budding daughter lesions is quite characteristic for progression of the infection in the abscess stage.

References

1. Schroth P et al. Advantage of magnetic resonance imaging in the diagnosis of cerebral infections. *Neuroradiology* 1987;29:120–126.
2. Brant-Zawadzki M et al. NMR imaging of experimental brain abscess: comparison with CT. *AJNR* 1983;4:250–253.
3. Salaki M et al. Fungal and yeast infections of the central nervous system: a clinical review. *Medicine* 1984;63:108–132.
4. Sze G. Infections and inflammatory diseases. In: Stark DD, Bradley WG, eds. *Magnetic resonance imaging.* St. Louis: C.V. Mosby Co., 1988;317–343.
5. Rosenbloom M et al. Decreased mortality from brain abscess since advent of computerized tomography. *J Neurosurg* 1978;49:658–668.
6. Enzman D et al. Experimental brain abscess evolution: computed tomographic and neuropathologic correlation. *Radiology* 1979;133:113–122.

Submitted by: D. Hinshaw, M.D., Loma Linda University, Loma Linda, California; Michael Brant-Zawadzki, M.D., Senior Editor.

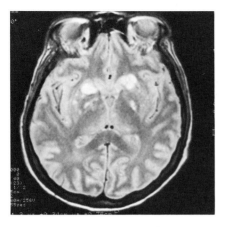

FIG. 12A. SE 3,000/40.

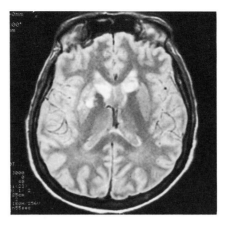

FIG. 12B. SE 3,000/40.

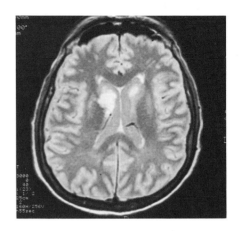

FIG. 12C. SE 3,000/40.

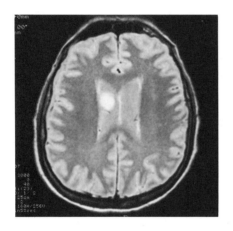

FIG. 12D. SE 3,000/40.

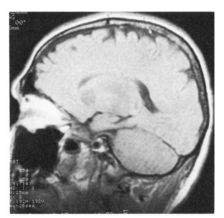

FIG. 12E. SE 850/20.

Clinical History

A 50-year-old male with altered mental status.

Findings

The T2-weighted axial (first echo) images depict multi-focal abnormalities within the basal ganglia. These consist of spherical and oval high signal lesions with mild-mass effect evident as indentation of the ventricular system (12A, 12D). The T1-weighted sagittal sequence (12E) shows the large lesion of the right caudate nucleus exhibiting well-circumscribed to low signal intensity characteristics. Thus, high water content is indicated by the combination of the T1- and T2-weighted sequences for this lesion.

This MRI picture is quite non-specific. However, several entities come to mind in the differential diagnosis.

Multiple basal ganglial infarcts are suggested, although this distribution is not typical as both right and left vascular territories are involved. Therefore, vasculitis is a possibility—as might be seen with meningitis or other causes of that entity. A relative lack of lesions elsewhere at the gray-white junction goes against the diagnosis of vasculitis. If the history of immune compromise were present (none in this case), the possibility of toxoplasmosis or other opportunistic infection might be raised. Lymphoma is also in the differential. Metastatic disease would be expected to show more in the way of mass effect and surrounding edema.

Diagnosis

Cryptococcosis.

Discussion

Cryptococcus neoformans has a worldwide distribution and is found in bird excreta, primarily that of pigeons, as well as in soil, especially in areas of avian habitation. Inhalation of the organism is the usual route of entry. The virulence and inoculum, as well as the adequacy of host defenses, determine primary patterns of disease. Cryptococcosis of the central nervous system manifests as either chronic meningitis, encephalitis, or mass lesions called *cryptococcomas*. Approximately 50% of patients have an underlying disease that limits host defenses; the others have no immune compromise. Chest lesions are associated in approximately 20% of the cases of central nervous system (CNS) cryptococcosis. Meningitis is the typical entity seen with CNS cryptococcosis. Spread up the prominent Virchow-Robin spaces in the basal ganglia accounts for the parenchymal involvement predominating these. The diagnosis generally is made based on cerebrospinal fluid (CSF) sampling. Positive India ink preparation of the fluid is the classic diagnostic finding. The MR picture shown here is that of cryptococcomas. In this patient, the infection led to the patient's demise, the disease proved pathologically in the brain.

References

1. Yoshikaw T et al. Management of central nervous system cryptococcosis. *West J Med* 1980;132:123–133.
2. Sze G et al. Infections and inflammatory diseases. In: Stark DD, Bradley WG, eds. *Magnetic resonance imaging.* St. Louis: C.V. Mosby Co., 1988;317–343.
3. Schroth H et al. Advantage of magnetic resonance imaging in the diagnosis of cerebral infections. *Neuroradiology* 1987;29:120–126.

Submitted by: Michael Brant-Zawadzki, M.D., Senior Editor.

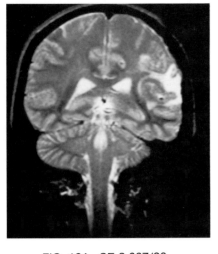

FIG. 13A. SE 2,667/80.

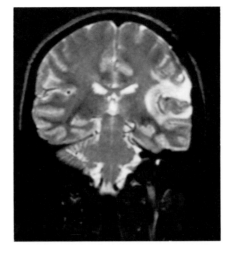

FIG. 13B. SE 2,667/80.

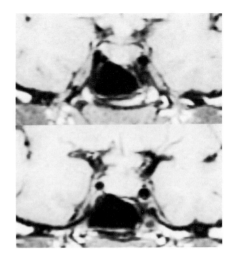

FIG. 13C. SE 800/25.

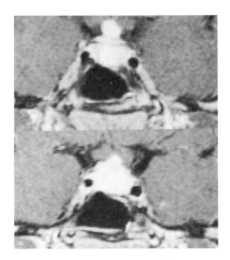

FIG. 13D. SE 600/25 with Gd-DTPA.

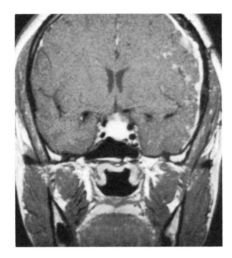

FIG. 13E. SE 600/25 with Gd-DTPA.

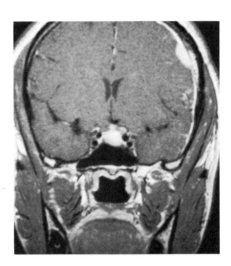

FIG. 13F. SE 600/25 with Gd-DTPA.

Clinical History

A 32-year-old female with headaches, diabetes insipidus.

Findings

T2-weighted coronal images (13A, 13B) show nonspecific white matter edema along the left temporal-parietal convexity. Cone down views of the suprasellar cistern suggest a soft tissue mass there on T1-weighted imaging in the coronal plane (13C). Contrast enhancement verifies the lesion in the suprasellar cistern and shows its intimate relationship to the pituitary stalk as well as suggestion of dural thickening of the diaphragma sella (13D). The more posterior coronal views verify dural-leptomeningeal abnormality along the left parietal-temporal convexity in the region of the vasogenic edema (13E, 13F).

Diagnosis

Intracranial sarcoidosis.

Discussion

Autopsy studies document an incidence of intracranial sarcoid in up to 14% of those patients with known sarcoidosis. Clinical neurologic manifestations will occur in approximately 5% of patients with systemic sarcoid. These may be the initial manifestation of the disease. Typically, subfrontal meningeal lesions are the hallmark of the disease on CT and/or MR imaging. Suprasellar/hypothalamic involvement is also seen and can produce diabetes insipidus. Leptomeningeal convexity lesions with marked white matter edema can also be found. Hydrocephalus will occur frequently. Hydrocephalus can be caused by periventricular inflammation, compression of the sylvian aqueduct, or simply the inflammation of the subarachnoid spaces. It should be noted that parenchymal disease can occur as multiple nodules within any part of the brain. This is felt to be the mechanism of the hypothalamic problem in this particular patient.

Differential diagnosis would include any chronic meningeal inflammatory process including infectious etiologies such as tuberculosis. Meningeal carcinomatosis is also in the differential. Eosinophilic granuloma could simulate the appearance of the suprasellar lesion in this case, but it would be less likely to involve the convexities.

References

1. Hayes SW, Sherman JL, Stern BJ. MR and CT evaluation of intracranial sarcoidosis. *AJNR* 1987;8:841–847.
2. Delany P. Neurological manifestation in sarcoidosis: review of the literature with a report of 23 cases. *Ann Intern Med* 1977;1987:336–345.
3. Ricker W, Clark M. Sarcoidosis, a clinical pathologic review of 300 cases, including 22 autopsies. *Am J Clin Pathol* 1949;19:725–749.

Submitted by: Wallace Peck, M.D., St. Joseph's Hospital, Orange, California; Michael Brant-Zawadzki, M.D., Senior Editor.

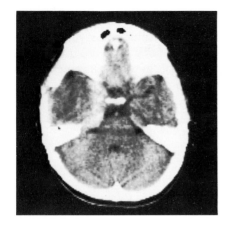

FIG. 14A. CT.

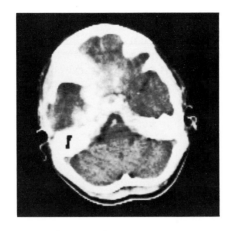

FIG. 14B. CT with contrast.

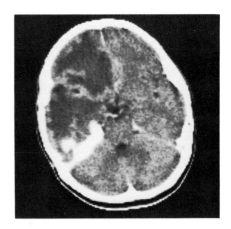

FIG. 14C. CT with contrast.

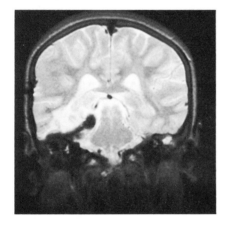

FIG. 14D. SE 2,800/80.

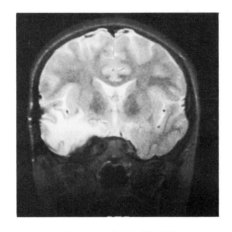

FIG. 14E. SE 2,800/80.

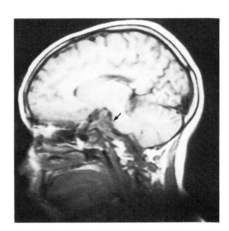

FIG. 14F. SE 600/20.

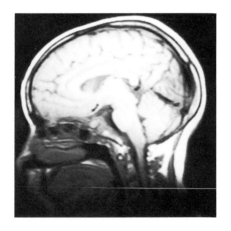

FIG. 14G. SE 600/20.

Clinical History

A young Mexican female with severe headaches, altered sensorium, fever, right-sided cranial palsy.

Findings

The CT scan before (14A) and after (14B) injection of intravenous contrast shows an inherently dense lesion at the base of the brain, which enhances homogeneously and is associated with marked vasogenic edema on the higher cuts (14C). The enhancement appears to be predominantly distributed along the basal meninges.

The MR scan [T2-weighted, coronal images (14D, 14E)] shows the region of the involved tentorial and basal middle fossa meninges as thickened, with preferential low signal intensity and corresponding vasogenic edema. The T1-weighted sagittal images show a shaggy appearance to the extra-axial space over the clivus and extending into the right middle fossa (14F, arrow; 14G).

Diagnosis

Tuberculous meningitis.

Discussion

Intracranial tuberculosis results from hematogenous spread from an evident or dormant primary focus of infection elsewhere. However, up to 30% of such cases have no prior or current evidence of extracranial infection. Central nervous system (CNS) tuberculosis presents most frequently as basilar meningitis, although tuberculomas also occur in the intra-axial space. A cerebritis may precede the development of frank tuberculous abscess in the brain.

In the meninges, a chronic inflammatory granulation tissue reaction occurs with vascular compromise, thus accompanying infarction may be seen and a picture of vasculitis, or large vessel occlusion, may be noted on angiograms. A hemorrhagic component to the exudate can occur and most likely is responsible for the hyperdensity on CT and the preferential low signal on T2-weighted images in this case.

The differential diagnosis with this MR appearance includes any cause of infectious or noninfectious inflammatory chronic meningeal process, as well as meningeal carcinomatosis. In general, meningioma en plaque incites much less vasogenic edema and shows a more homogeneous sheet-like appearance but is also in the differential diagnosis.

References

1. Gupta R, Jena A, Sharma A, et al. MR imaging of intracranial tuberculomas. *J Comput Assist Tomogr* 1988;12:280–285.
2. Dasturd K, Lalitha V, Udani P, et al. The brain and meninges in tuberculomatous meningitis—gross pathology in 100 cases and pathogenesis. *Neurology* (India) 1970;18:86–100.
3. Bhargava S, Gupta A, Tandon P. Tuberculous meningitis: a CT study. *Br J Radiol* 1982;55:189–196.

Submitted by: Wallace Peck, M.D., St. Joseph's Hospital, Orange, California; Michael Brant-Zawadzki, M.D., Senior Editor.

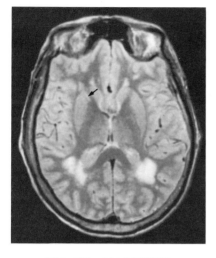

FIG. 15A. SE 3,000/40.

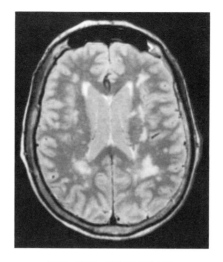

FIG. 15B. SE 3,000/40.

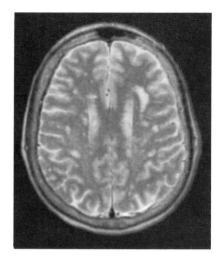

FIG. 15C. SE 3,000/80.

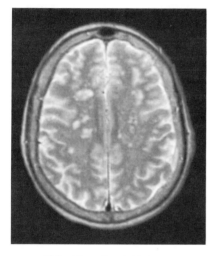

FIG. 15D. SE 3,000/80.

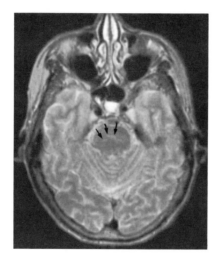

FIG. 15E. SE 3,000/40.

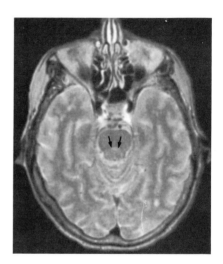

FIG. 15F. SE 3,000/80.

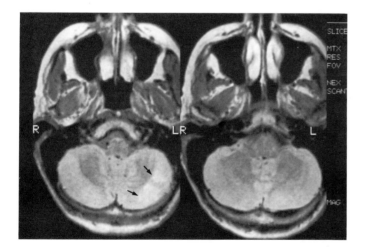

FIG. 15G. SE 3,000/40.

Clinical History

A 74-year-old female with long-standing headaches.

Findings

Axial 5 mm T2-W (SE 3,000/40 and 80 msec) images are presented. There are extensive multiple 1–2 cm foci of increased signal intensity in the periventricular white matter bilaterally (15A–15C). These lesions are relatively symmetrical, spare the subependymal white matter, and are more prominent in the frontal and occipital regions, predominantly involving the white matter of the corona radiata and centrum semiovale. Apart from a single lesion in the anterior limb of the right internal capsule, the basal ganglia are spared (15A). There are also poorly defined, transversely-oriented fine bands of increased signal involving the central and upper pons (15E, 15F). There is a cortically based region of increased signal intensity involving the posterior-inferior left cerebellar hemisphere. Mucous is noted in the sphenoid sinus.

Diagnosis

Deep white matter infarction; inferior left cerebellar infarct.

Discussion

Focal and confluent areas of periventricular hyperintensity on T2-weighted images have been reported on MR images from between 30% and 60% of patients over the age of 60 years (1–4). These lesions are related to microangiopathy (arteriolar disease) affecting the small, penetrating end arteries. Territories supplied by these vessels are particularly susceptible to ischemic disease: the deep cerebral white matter (via medullary arteries), the caudate, anterior limb of the internal capsule, putamen, globus pallidus (lenticulostriate arteries), thalamus (thalamogeniculate end arteries), posterior limb of the internal capsule (anterior choroidal artery), and the pons (long, perforating branches of basilar artery). Superficial (subcortical) cerebral white matter and the arcuate "u" fibers are generally spared due to their dual vascular supply. There are three periventricular boundary zones between penetrating vessels involving the anterior corpus callosum and pons, the deep white matter adjacent to the atrium and occipital horn, and the deep white matter adjacent to the frontal horns. These anatomic features help to explain the preponderance of these lesions in the occipito-frontal regions.

The underlying pathology shows central areas of true infarction surrounded by much larger areas of gliosis. If there are central areas of cavitation, then changes may be present on T1-weighted images. Other pathologically recognized lesions include myelin pallor, axonal loss, perivascular demyelination, and gliosis. Despite the extensive appearance of these lesions, they are often found in patients without neurological deficits. Conversely, a clinically dementing illness in a patient with even extensive periventricular hyperintensity does not confirm the diagnosis of vascular dementia. However, the absence of multiple white matter abnormalities in the atrophic brain in a demented individual strongly favors the diagnosis of a primary dementia such as Alzheimer's disease.

Although in this case the brainstem findings are subtle, ill-defined transverse lesions involving the central portion of the pons sparing the medulla and midbrain are often seen in association with the supratentorial periventricular abnormalities in patients without any clinical evidence of brainstem dysfunction. Their intensity often parallels the severity of the disease within the brain. Again these lesions represent a spectrum that includes loss of myelin, astrocytic proliferation, and patchy infarction due to lipohyalinosis of penetrating vessels arising from the basilar artery.

References

1. Marshall BG, Bradley WG, Marshall CE, et al. Deep white matter infarction: correlation of MR imaging and histopathological findings. *Radiology* 1988;167:517–522.
2. Braffman BH, Zimmerman RA, Trojanowski JQ, et al. Brain MR: pathological correlation with gross and histopathology. White matter foci in the elderly. *AJNR* 1988;9:629–636.
3. Drayer BP. MR imaging of the aging brain, part I: normal findings. *Radiology* 1988;166:785–796.
4. Salomon A, Yeates AE, Burger PC, et al. Subcortical arteriosclerotic encephalopathy: brainstem findings with MR imaging. *Radiology* 1988;165:625–629.

Submitted by: Stephen J. Davis, M.D. and Louis M. Teresi, M.D., Huntington Medical Research Institutes, Pasadena, California; William G. Bradley, Jr., M.D., Ph.D., Senior Editor.

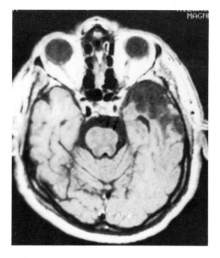

FIG. 16A. SE 700/25 with Gd-DTPA.

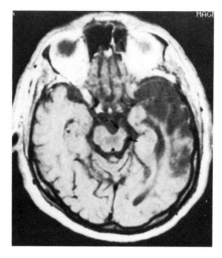

FIG. 16B. SE 700/25 with Gd-DTPA.

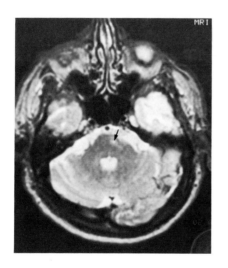

FIG. 16C. SE 2,900/90.

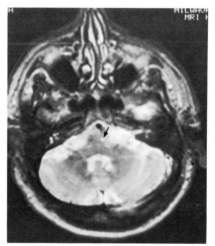

FIG. 16D. SE 2,900/90.

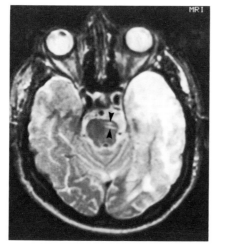

FIG. 16E. SE 2,900/90.

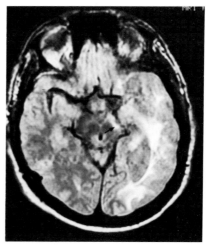

FIG. 16F. SE 2,900/40.

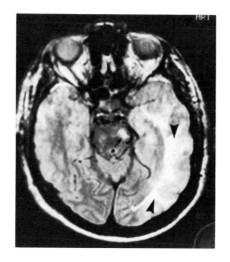

FIG. 16G. SE 2,900/40.

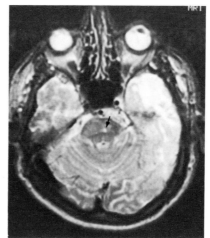

FIG. 16H. SE 2,900/90.

Clinical History

A 73-year-old male with 7-year history of right hemiparesis.

Findings

Axial 5 mm T2-W (SE 2,900/40 and 90) and axial 5 mm T1-W (SE 700/25) images are presented.

There is a very large, cortically-based lesion involving the left temporal, parietal, and frontal lobes, insular cortex, and basal ganglia. This lesion involves the entire middle cerebral artery territory on this side (16B, 16G, 16I–16K). The lesion shows marked T1 and T2 lengthening with near-cerebrospinal fluid (CSF) intensity on both T1- and T2-weighted sequences (16I, 16J, arrows). At the margin of this lesion and adjacent normal brain, there is a marked irregular rim of high signal intensity on the first echo of the long TR sequence (16G, 16K, arrowheads). There is accompanying dilatation of the left lateral ventricle.

There is atrophy of the left cerebral peduncle in the midbrain and of the left side of the belly of the pons (16A, 16B, arrows). There is a linear increased signal intensity seen on the T2-weighted sequences in the expected position of the left corticospinal tract (16C, 16D, 16F–16H, arrows). Gyriform low signal intensity is present in the residual cortex overlying the infarct (16J, arrows) (due to hemosiderin).

There is a small, wedge-shaped, cortically-based region of high signal intensity in the lateral right parietal lobe, likely to represent a small cortical infarct. There are several punctate areas of increased signal intensity in the deep white matter of the right cerebral hemisphere due to deep white matter infarction.

Diagnosis

Chronic extensive infarction in the distribution of the left middle cerebral artery with Wallerian degeneration of the left corticospinal tract; small right cortical infarct; mild deep white matter infarction.

Discussion

Wallerian degeneration involves degeneration of axons and the myelin sheaths distal to a site of proximal axonal or cell body neural injury. The degeneration follows the usual direction of nerve conduction, away from the cell body. This degeneration results in an increase in extracellular water, causing prolongation of T1 and T2 relaxation times. Although axonal degeneration occurs quickly, demyelination is slower and may take six months. The corticospinal tract arises from cell bodies in the cerebral cortex and descends through the corona radiata, posterior limb of the internal capsule and cerebral peduncles into the basis pontis where the fibers are separated by transverse pontine fascicles. The fibers descend through the pyramids anteriorly in the medulla before decussating in the lower medulla to travel in the contralateral lateral corticospinal tract of the spinal cord. The pontine separation is shown in Figure 16E (black arrowheads). Although cerebral infarction is the most common associated disorder, neoplasms or demyelinating or traumatic lesions can also give rise to Wallerian degeneration.

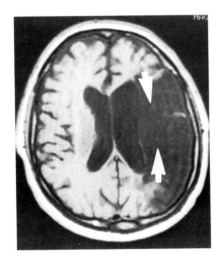

FIG. 16I. SE 700/75.

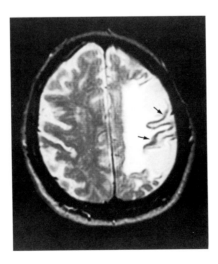

FIG. 16J. SE 2,900/90.

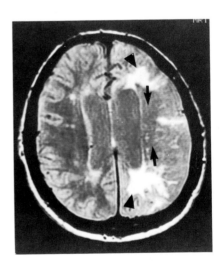

FIG. 16K. SE 2,900/40.

34

Reference

1. Kuhn MJ, Johnson KA, Davis KR. Wallerian degeneration: evaluation with MR imaging. *Radiology* 1988;168:199.

Submitted by: Stephen J. Davis, M.D. and Louis M. Teresi, M.D., Huntington Medical Research Institutes, Pasadena, California; William G. Bradley, Jr., M.D., Ph.D., Senior Editor.

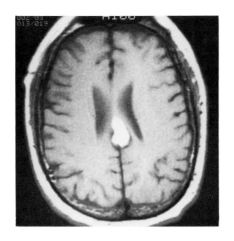

FIG. 17A. SE 800/20.

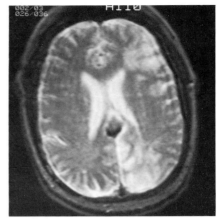

FIG. 17B. SE 2,800/20.

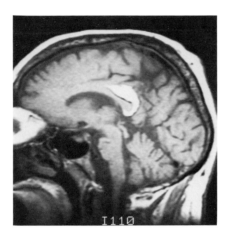

FIG. 17C. SE 600/20.

Clinical History

A 66-year-old male with sudden onset of visual loss, right body weakness, suspected cerebrovascular accident.

Findings

T1-weighted axial image (17A) shows a focus of high signal intensity in the posterior midline. Given the history, a bleed here might be suspected. The T2-weighted image (partly degraded due to patient motion) shows the signal intensity of the lesion to have faded, with particularly prominent low signal intensity posteriorly at the border of the lesion (17B). In addition, geographic cortical high signal intensity is seen in the left high occipital pole, as well as in the left frontal parietal cortex. The T1-weighted sagittal image (17C) verifies the midline lesion to be closely associated with the corpus callosum.

Diagnosis

Acute left hemispheric infarct: incidental corpus callosum lipoma (simulating bleed).

Discussion

The clinical history here is that of a stroke. Although the midline lesion might be assumed to represent hemorrhage initially, the fading of signal from the T1- through the T2-weighted image would be somewhat atypical for blood (although occasionally, a combination of intracellular methemoglobin and methemoglobin in solution could produce such a change). With sufficient methemoglobin formation to produce the high signal intensity on T1-weighted images, persistent high signal would be expected on the T2-weighted image (methemoglobin in solution should be bright on T2-weighted images as well). The curvilinear nature of the lesion on the sagittal T1-weighted image and the close application of it to the corpus callosum are quite typical for a midline corpus callosum lipoma—a developmental incidental finding.

The gyriform high signal of the gray matter in the posterior parietal-occipital cortex as well as in the left frontal-parietal region is quite typical for acute infarction (in this case less than two days old), which explains the patient's symptoms. No evidence of hemorrhage in the region of infarction is present on either the T2- or the T1-weighted image. In general, hemorrhagic stroke represents secondary conversion of ischemic infarction by hemorrhage due to perfusion "break through." Such conversion is manifest by magnetic susceptibility effects within the otherwise high signal of the infarcted region.

References

1. Brant-Zawadzki M et al. MR imaging and spectroscopy in clinical and experimental cerebral ischemia: a review. *AJNR* 1987;8:39–48.
2. Sipponen J. Visualization of brain infarction with nuclear magnetic resonance imaging. *Neuroradiology* 1984;26:387–391.
3. Zettner W et al. Lipoma of the corpus callosum. *J Neuropathol Exp Neurol* 1960;19:305–309.

Submitted by: Michael Brant-Zawadzki, M.D., Senior Editor.

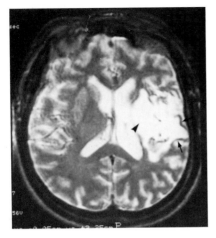

FIG. 18A. SE 3,000/100.

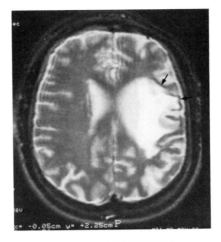

FIG. 18B. SE 3,000/100.

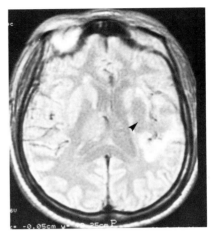

FIG. 18C. SE 3,000/25.

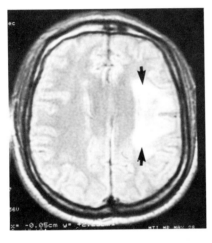

FIG. 18D. SE 3,000/25.

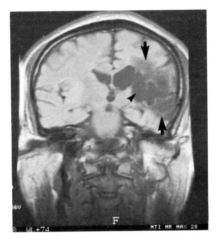

FIG. 18E. SE 1,000/25.

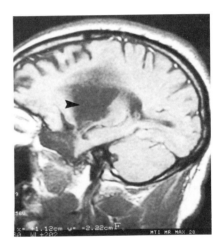

FIG. 18F. SE 700/25.

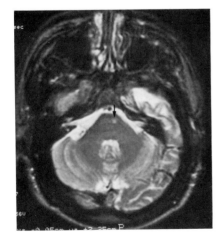

FIG. 18G. SE 3,000/100.

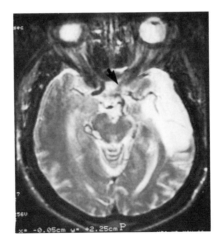

FIG. 18H. SE 3,000/100.

Clinical History

A 55-year-old male with right hemiparesis for six years.

Findings

Axial 5 mm T2-W (SE 3,000/25 and 100), sagittal 5 mm T1-W (SE 700/25), and coronal 10 mm T1-W (SE 1,000/25) images are presented.

There is a large cortically-based lesion involving the anterior temporal lobe, insular cortex, putamen, caudate, and internal capsule (18A–18F). This lesion has large central components that are isointense with CSF on all sequences (18A, 18C, 18E, 18F, arrowheads) surrounded by regions of increased signal intensity, best seen on the first echo of the long TR sequence (18C, arrowhead). This zone is also seen on the short TR sequence as intermediate signal intensity between brain and CSF (18E, arrows). Residual cortex seen supralaterally shows evidence of T2 shortening with low signal seen in this region on the most T2-weighted sequence (18A, 18B, arrows). There is dilatation of the ipsilateral lateral ventricle and adjacent cortical sulci. There is atrophy of the left cerebellar peduncle and left side of the pons, and there is a 3 mm longitudinal band of increased signal traversing the anterior aspect of the right side of the pons extending anteriorly into the medulla, in the expected position of the corticospinal tract (18G, arrows).

No flow void is seen in the left internal carotid artery (18H, arrow).

Diagnosis

Occlusion of the left internal carotid artery with chronic infarction involving the left middle cerebral artery territory and Wallerian degeneration of the left corticospinal tract.

Discussion

This chronic infarct shows areas of both macrocystic and microcystic encephalomalacia on moderately T2-weighted images. Two zones are seen: one of hyperintensity between the normal brain and the more central zone of CSF intensity. The peripheral region corresponds to smaller cystic spaces seen microscopically and is thus termed *microcystic encephalomalacia,* or *gliosis.* The largest cystic spaces (which follow the intensity of CSF) are termed *macrocystic encephalomalacia.* These cavities result from liquefactive necrosis and may be seen in any injury resulting in brain necrosis. The different MR characteristics of microcystic and macrocystic encephalomalacia are due to different environments of the water in the brain. Small cysts in the microcystic form provide a relatively large surface area attracting the water molecules into hydration layers, resulting in T1 shortening relative to CSF, and, therefore, increased signal intensity. In the macrocystic form, the water is in the bulk phase and thus has a similar appearance to CSF. This pattern is also seen following trauma, surgery, or other forms of brain injury.

The cortical ribbon of T2 shortening is called *superficial siderosis* and is due to residual hemosiderin staining from petechial hemorrhage associated with the infarction. Although this is a characteristic sequella of hemorrhagic infarctions that typically occur in the middle cerebral artery distribution, it may also be seen in "bland infarctions" (by CT) where microscopic petechial hemorrhage is seen pathologically in up to 40% of cases.

Reference

1. Bradley WG. Pathophysiologic correlates of signal alterations. In: Brant-Zawadzki M, Norman D, eds. *Magnetic resonance imaging of the central nervous system.* New York: Raven Press, 1987;23–42.

Submitted by: Stephen J. Davis, M.D. and Louis M. Teresi, M.D., Huntington Medical Research Institutes, Pasadena, California; William G. Bradley, Jr., M.D., Ph.D., Senior Editor.

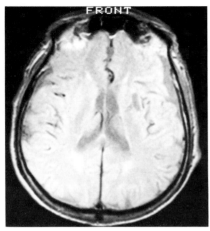
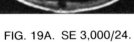
FIG. 19A. SE 3,000/24.

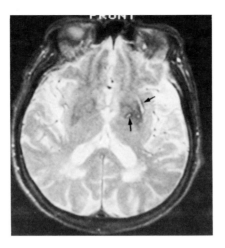
FIG. 19B. SE 3,000/90.

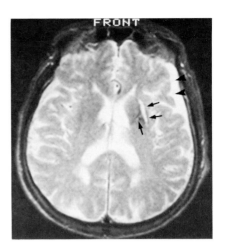
FIG. 19C. SE 3,000/90.

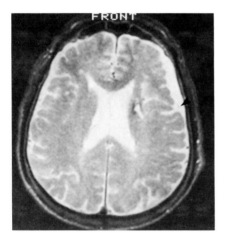
FIG. 19D. SE 3,000/90.

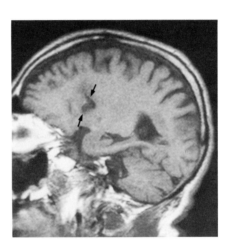
FIG. 19E. SE 500/18.

Clinical History

An 81-year-old hypertensive male with history of previous sudden onset of severe right hemiparesis that had partially resolved.

Findings

Axial 6 mm T2-W (SE 3,000/24 and 90) and sagittal 6 mm T1-W (SE 500/18) images are presented.

There is a slit-like defect within the lateral aspect of the left putamen measuring 2 cm in the anteroposterior dimension and 5 mm laterally that has internal signal characteristics similar to CSF (19A–19E), but that is surrounded on the more heavily T2-weighted sequences by a rim of low signal intensity (19C, black arrows). There are several punctate adjacent lesions in the globus pallidus (19B), which are seen to communicate with the previously described lesion superiorly. These extend into the internal capsule and corona radiata.

There are multiple focal areas of increased signal intensity within the deep white matter bilaterally. A small extra-axial CSF collection is noted overlying the lateral aspect of the left frontal lobe, evidenced by displacement of the cortical veins centrally (19C, 19D, arrowheads) and focal effacement of the cortical sulci. This measures 1 cm in width and extends over a length of approximately 5 cm.

Diagnosis

Previous putaminal hypertensive hemorrhage; small left subdural hygroma; deep white matter infarction.

Discussion

Hypertensive intracerebral hemorrhage is often catastrophic—75% of patients dying in the first 30 days. If the patient survives the initial ictus, then the prognosis is relatively good as the hematoma dissects along white matter tracts and causes symptoms by mass effect rather than by causing direct localized infarction. Rebleeding is unusual at the same site. The putamen is a classic site for a hypertensive bleed and characteristically produces slit-like defects stained with hemosiderin. Other common sites of hypertensive hemorrhage include the thalamus, the pons, and the cerebellum. In this case, the hemosiderin rim causes T2 shortening with a rim of low signal intensity being produced on the T2-weighted images. The shape of the lesion is characteristic of hypertensive slit hemorrhage.

The subdural hemorrhage collection is chronic and represents either a chronic hematoma or subdural hygroma.

Reference

1. Bradley WG. Hemorrhage and vascular abnormalities. In: Bradley WG, Bydder GM. *MRI atlas of the brain.* London: Martin Dunitz, 1990; 201–264.

Submitted by: Stephen J. Davis, M.D. and Louis M. Teresi, M.D., Huntington Medical Research Institutes, Pasadena, California; William G. Bradley, Jr., M.D., Ph.D., Senior Editor.

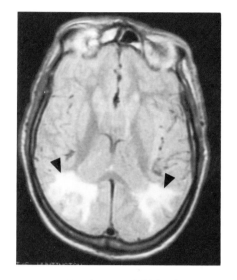

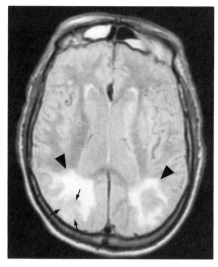

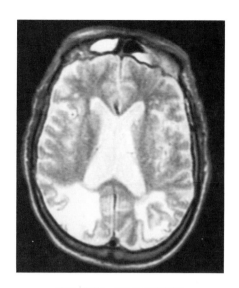

FIG. 20A. SE 3,000/40.

FIG. 20B. SE 3,000/40.

FIG. 20C. SE 3,000/80.

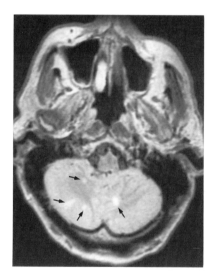

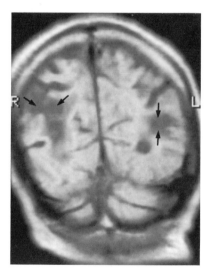

FIG. 20D. SE 3,000/40.

FIG. 20E. SE 1,000/30.

Clinical History

A 77-year-old male with dementia, depression, and seizures.

Findings

Axial 5 mm T2-W (SE 3,000/40 and 80) and coronal 10 mm T1-W (SE 1,000/30) images are presented.

There are hyperintense, wedge-shaped lesions involving the junctions of the parietal and occipital lobes bilaterally, more marked on the right, seen on the T2-weighted sequences (20A–20C). These lesions extend from the posterior aspect of the atria of both lateral ventricles to the cortex and show decreased signal intensity on the T1-weighted images (20D). There is evidence of peripheral "macrocystic encephalomalacia," where the intensity of the lesion follows that of CSF (20B, 20E, black arrows), separated from the normal brain by a large area of microcystic encephalomalacia (gliosis) characterized by high signal intensity on the first echo of the T2-weighted sequence (20A, 20B, arrowheads). No abnormality of the cerebral vasculature is seen.

There are several small 3–7 mm diameter lesions in the cerebellar hemispheres bilaterally (20D, arrows). These lesions are distributed at the junction of the deep cerebellar white matter and the overlying cerebellar cortex.

There are scattered punctate foci of increased signal intensity in the deep white matter bilaterally; 1 cm lesion is present in the periventricular left corona radiata. A retention cyst is noted in the right maxillary sinus and in the lateral recess of the left sphenoid sinus, and there is mucosal thickening in the maxillary, ethmoid, and frontal sinuses bilaterally.

Diagnosis

Bilateral watershed infarcts between the distributions of the middle and posterior cerebral arteries, more marked on the right; bilateral cerebellar watershed infarcts; mild deep white-matter ischemia/infarction; paranasal sinus disease.

Discussion

Watershed or hemodynamic infarction occurs when there is temporary underperfusion of the brain, usually in older patients with hypertension, who may also have stenoses in major cerebral arteries and who develop underperfusion from either a cardiac arrhythmia or hypotensive episode. These patients suffer underperfusion and resultant hemodynamic infarction at the junctions of the anterior, middle and posterior cerebral artery circulations that have the lowest perfusion pressures, being terminal areas of supply of these arteries. The parietal-occipital borders are the most susceptible to this injury. The ischemic injury may remain localized to the cortex, referred to as laminar necrosis, involving the third, fifth, or sixth cortical layers that are particularly vulnerable. If the ischemic insult is more severe, more layers along with the underlying white matter are involved. It may be hemorrhagic in nature once reperfusion of the damaged area occurs.

Watershed infarction may also occur in the cerebellum, usually in the boundary between the areas supplied by the superior cerebellar and the posterior inferior cerebellar arteries, or at the lateral angle of the cerebellum between the posterior-inferior cerebellar artery (PICA), superior cerebellar, and anterior-inferior cerebellar artery (AICA) territories. Small cortical watershed infarcts must be differentiated from enlargement of the great horizontal fissure. The infarcts seen in this patient are also watershed infarcts at the border zone between the penetrating branches of the PICA, superior cerebral artery (SCA), and AICA. These lesions typically occur in the mid-cerebellar white matter or gray-white matter junction.

References

1. Gado MH. Supratentorial anatomy. In: Stark DD, Bradley WG, eds. *Magnetic resonance imaging.* St. Louis: The C. V. Mosby Company, 1988:269–298.
2. Goldberg HI. Hemodynamic infarction. In: Lee SH, Rao KCVG, eds. *Cranial computed tomography.* New York: McGraw Hill, 1987;610–616.
3. Savoiardo M, Bracchi M, Passerini A, et al. The vascular territories in the cerebellum and brainstem: CT and MR study. *AJNR* 1987;8:199.

Submitted by: Stephen J. Davis, M.D. and Louis M. Teresi, M.D., Huntington Medical Research Institutes, Pasadena, California; William G. Bradley, Jr., M.D., Ph.D., Senior Editor.

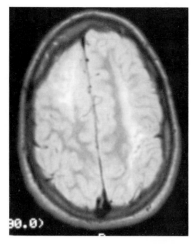

FIG. 21A. SE 3,000/30.

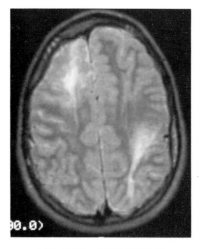

FIG. 21B. SE 3,000/75.

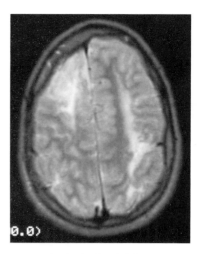

FIG. 21C. SE 3,000/75.

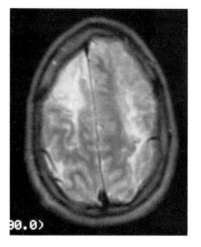

FIG. 21D. SE 3,000/75.

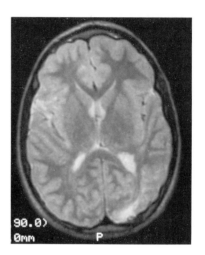

FIG. 21E. SE 3,000/75.

Clinical History

A 12-year-old boy with birth asphyxia, requiring intensive neonatal care for two weeks with subsequent seizure disorder and mild development delay.

Findings

Axial 5 mm T2-W (SE 3,000/30 and 75) images are presented.

There are high signal intensity zones involving the subcortical white matter of both cerebral hemispheres distributed linearly in the watershed between the distribution of the anterior cerebral artery parasagittal cortical strips and the cerebral convexity supplied by the middle cerebral artery (21A–21D). The left-sided lesion extends posteroinferiorly into the parieto-occipital junctional region between the distribution of the left posterior and middle cerebral arteries (21E).

Diagnosis

Bilateral watershed infarcts between the distributions of the anterior and middle cerebral arteries, and on the left also between the middle and posterior cerebral arteries.

Discussion

The distribution of these lesions is typical of the watershed distribution between the anterior and middle cerebral arteries. Watershed infarction most often occurs between the middle and posterior artery circulations, but the distribution shown here is the second most frequent seen.

Reference

1. Goldberg HI. Hemodynamic infarction. In: Lee SH, Rao KCVG, eds. *Cranial computed tomography.* New York: McGraw Hill, 1987;610–616.

Submitted by: Stephen J. Davis, M.D. and Louis M. Teresi, M.D., Huntington Medical Research Institutes, Pasadena, California; William G. Bradley, Jr., M.D., Ph.D., Senior Editor.

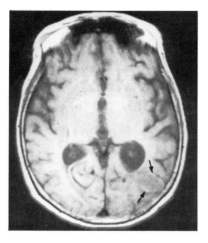
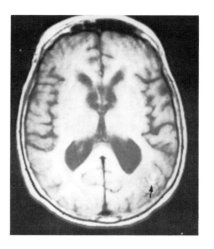
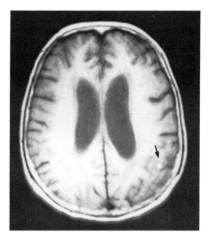

FIG. 22A. SE 600/20. FIG. 22B. SE 600/20. FIG. 22C. SE 600/20.

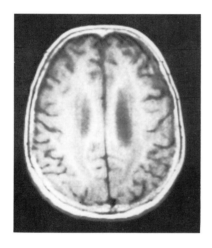
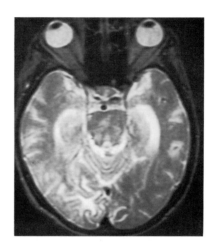

FIG. 22D. SE 600/20. FIG. 22E. SE 2,800/80.

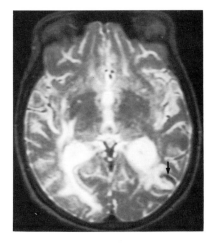

FIG. 22F. SE 2,800/80.

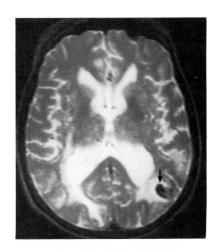

FIG. 22G. SE 2,800/80.

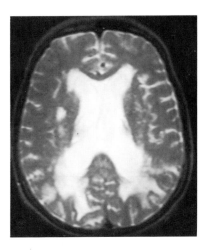

FIG. 22H. SE 2,800/80.

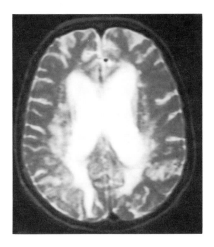

FIG. 22I. SE 2,800/80.

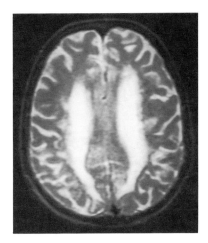

FIG. 22J. SE 2,800/80.

47

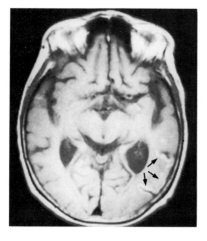
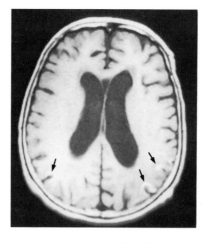
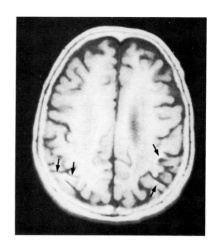

FIG. 22K. SE 600/20.   FIG. 22L. SE 600/20.   FIG. 22M. SE 600/20.

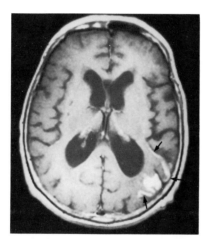
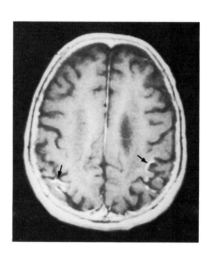

FIG. 22N. SE 600/20 with Gd-DTPA.   FIG. 22O. SE 600/20 with Gd-DTPA.

Clinical History

A 69-year-old woman with confusion for several days prior to the scan.

48

Findings

Two studies are presented: the first taken at the time of presentation and the second taken three weeks later.

From the first study, axial 5 mm T1-W (SE 600/20) and axial 5 mm T2-W (SE 2,800/80) images are presented. On the T1-weighted images, in the posterolateral aspect of the left temporal lobe and inferior parietal lobe, there are multiple punctate and linear foci of increased signal intensity within the cerebral cortex (22A–22C, black arrows). There is some ill-defined decrease in signal intensity in the underlying white matter. On the T2-weighted images, there are similarly distributed linear hypointensities (22F, 22G, black arrows) with less well-defined increased signal extending into the subjacent white matter. There are patchy regions of cortical increased signal intensity involving the cortex and subcortical white matter in the posterior left temporal and parietal lobes (22G, 22I, 22J) and in the posterior right parietal lobe at the parieto-occipital junction (22G, 22I). There are scattered foci of increased signal intensity in the deep white matter bilaterally and in the pons.

The second sequence of films also includes 5 mm T1-W (SE 600/20) images before and after Gadolinium (3 weeks later). On the pre-Gadolinium study, there is now more extensive gyriform increased signal intensity involving the cortex of the left posterior temporal (22K) and parietal (22L, 22M) lobes. There are less marked but similar changes involving the right posterior parietal lobe. Following Gadolinium administration, extensive gyriform contrast enhancement is seen in the regions of the previously mentioned T1 shortening (22N, 22O, black arrows).

Diagnosis

Bilateral subacute hemorrhagic cortical infarcts.

Discussion

Hemorrhagic infarction is usually due to high-pressure reperfusion of infarcted brain and most often occurs in the clinical context of embolic infarction where reperfusion occurs after fragmentation and lysis of the embolus. Hemorrhagic infarction may also occur in atherosclerotic thrombotic infarcts in patients with coagulation disorders or those on anticoagulant therapy. It is also seen in venous infarction and watershed infarction. Small areas of petechial hemorrhage commonly occur pathologically in the periphery of otherwise bland infarcts.

The gyriform hypointensity shown in the initial study on the T2-weighted sequence is caused by intracellular deoxyhemoglobin or methemoglobin, causing T2 shortening. This is evidence of acute or early subacute hemorrhage. The accompanying gyriform increased signal on the T1-weighted image is due to methemoglobin formation (causing T1 shortening), indicating that there are at least some early subacute components of the hemorrhage.

Hemorrhagic cortical infarctions tend to occur in watershed regions and may occur at the margin of bland cortical infarctions. They have a predilection for deeper cortical layers and the deepest gyral folds (22L, black arrows). The sequence of changes in the signal characteristics of the blood parallels other regions. However, T2 shortening due to deoxyhemoglobin in the cortical zone is usually less marked than in deeper parenchymal hematomas, as the higher local oxygen tension and pH are secondary to the hyperemia of early vascular recanalization. Luxury perfusion lowers the concentration of intracellular deoxyhemoglobin and therefore decreases the relative T2 shortening. The gyriform cortical distribution of the intracellular methemoglobin and deoxyhemoglobin particularly in the depths of the cerebral sulci as seen in this case is characteristic of hemorrhagic cortical infarction. The distribution in this patient suggests that watershed infarction secondary to hypoperfusion is likely to be the cause. Most hemorrhagic infarctions are secondary to cerebral emboli and classically occur in the distribution of the middle cerebral artery. Cerebral emboli could, therefore, not be excluded in this case.

Reference

1. Hecht-Leavitt C, Gomori J, Grossman RI, et al. High field MRI of hemorrhagic cortical infarction. *AJNR* 1986;7:581–586.

Submitted by: Stephen J. Davis, M.D. and Louis M. Teresi, M.D., Huntington Medical Research Institutes, Pasadena, California; William G. Bradley, Jr., M.D., Ph.D., Senior Editor.

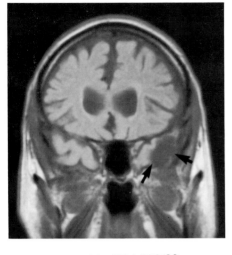

FIG. 23A. SE 1,000/30.

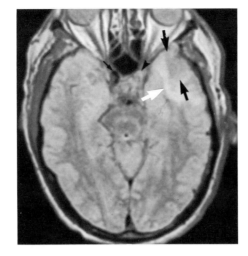

FIG. 23B. SE 3,000/30.

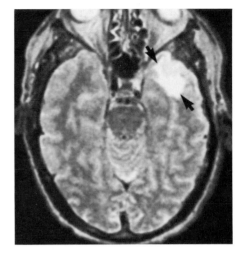

FIG. 23C. SE 3,000/80.

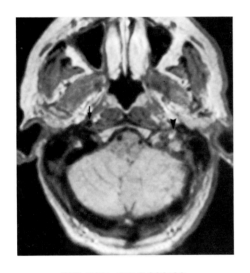

FIG. 23D. SE 3,000/30.

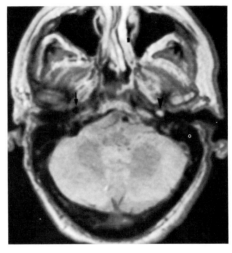

FIG. 23E. SE 3,000/30.

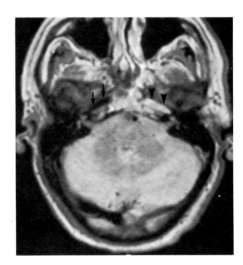

FIG. 23F. SE 3,000/30.

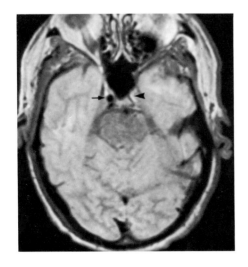

FIG. 23G. SE 3,000/30.

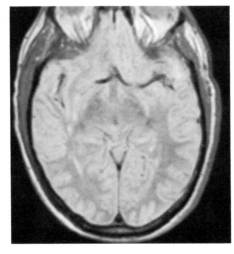

FIG. 23H. SE 3,000/30.

Clinical History

A 70-year-old male with speech difficulty for six months. Previous right carotid endarterectomy.

Findings

Axial 5 mm T2-W (SE 3,000/30 and 80) and coronal 10 mm T1-W (SE 1,000/30) images are presented.

There is an old infarct involving the left temporal tip that has resulted in macrocystic encephalomalacia, evidenced by focal atrophy with marked T1 and T2 lengthening (23A–23C, large black arrows). There is accompanying dilatation of the adjacent cerebral sulci and a peripheral zone of surrounding increased signal seen best on the first echo of the long TR sequence (23B, white arrow), representing microcystic encephalomalacia or "gliosis." (The high signal is due to T1 shortening from the hydration layer water effect of the multiple small cysts). The normal flow void of the left internal carotid artery is absent, being replaced by moderately high signal intensity throughout its length (arrowheads). [Compare this to the normal flow void in the right internal carotid artery (23B; 23D–23G, small black arrows).] There is no evidence of increased signal on the second echo image to suggest even-echo rephasing and flow. A normal flow void is reestablished in the left middle cerebral artery, presumably via circle of Willis collaterals (23H).

There are scattered punctate foci of high signal intensity in the deep white matter bilaterally.

Diagnosis

Chronic right temporal lobe infarct with macrocystic encephalomalacia; thrombosis or exceedingly slow flow through the right internal carotid artery.

Discussion

One of the advantages of MR when compared to CT in the assessment of stroke is the ability to evaluate the intracranial vasculature. The high signal seen throughout the length of the internal carotid artery on spin echo imaging is due to either thrombosis or exceedingly slow flow, as stationary blood has a long T2. It is not currently possible to positively differentiate these two conditions using routine spin echo imaging, although this may be achievable using phase imaging. Single slice gradient echo and MR angiography techniques may be useful in selected cases, although there is still difficulty in differentiating increases in signal due to thrombus from flow effects. Further evaluation using either Doppler ultrasound or, if clinically indicated, traditional angiography may be required to differentiate complete thrombosis from slow flow occurring beyond a high grade stenosis, and therefore to distinguish a potentially surgical lesion from complete occlusion.

Reference

1. Bradley WG. Pathophysiologic correlates of signal alterations. In: Brant-Zawadzki M, Norman D, eds. *Magnetic resonance imaging of the central nervous system.* New York: Raven Press. 1987;23–42.

Submitted by: Stephen J. Davis, M.D. and Louis M. Teresi, M.D., Huntington Medical Research Institutes, Pasadena, California; William G. Bradley, Jr., M.D., Ph.D., Senior Editor.

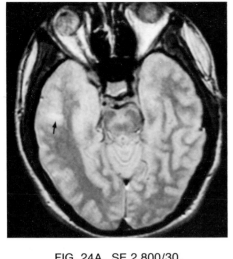

FIG. 24A. SE 2,800/30.

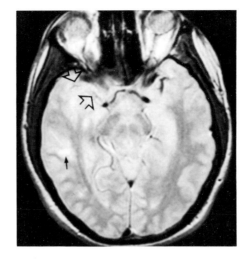

FIG. 24B. SE 2,800/30.

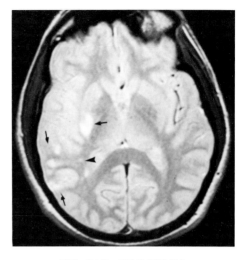

FIG. 24C. SE 2,800/30.

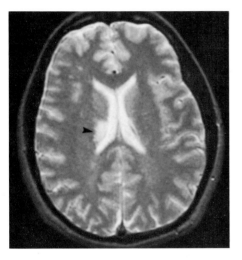

FIG. 24D. SE 2,800/80.

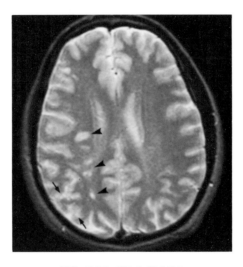

FIG. 24E. SE 2,800/80.

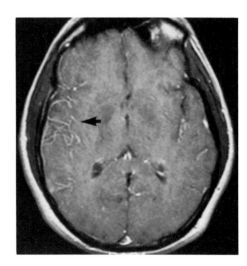

FIG. 24F. SE 700/30 with Gd-DTPA.

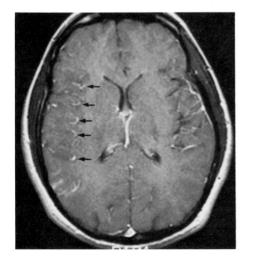

FIG. 24G. SE 700/30 with Gd-DTPA.

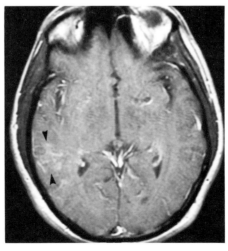

FIG. 24H. SE 700/30 with Gd-DTPA.

Clinical History

A 32-year-old male with a six-week history of intermittent left hand dysfunction.

Findings

Axial 5 mm T2-W (SE 2,800/30 and 80) and axial 5 mm Gd-DTPA enhanced T1-W (SE 700/30) images are presented.

There are multiple focal lesions in the right cerebral hemisphere. These lesions involve both the cortical gray matter and the basal ganglia (black arrows), and the intervening deep white matter (24A, 24B, small black arrows; 24C–24E, arrowheads). All lesions are distributed in the territory of the right middle cerebral artery, the lumen of which is not clearly visualized, although an outline of this vessel can be seen (24B, open arrows).

Following Gadolinium enhancement, multiple small serpiginous vessels are seen in the right sylvian fissure (24F, 24G, arrows). There is patchy contrast enhancement posteriorly in the right temporal cortex (24H, arrowheads).

Diagnosis

Cerebral infarction due to right middle cerebral artery occlusion.

Discussion

The distribution of all of these lesions in the vascular territory of the right middle cerebral artery raises the suspicion of a vascular etiology. This is heightened by involvement of the cortex, the basal ganglia, and the interposed white matter—cortical involvement being typical of arterial occlusive disease. The diagnosis is confirmed by the absence of the flow void in the right middle cerebral artery, emphasizing the value of MR imaging in this respect. The serpiginous vessels seen in the right sylvian fissure represent collateral circulation established by the anterior cerebral artery circulation with retrograde filling of the middle cerebral artery branches in the sylvian fissure. The symmetrical pattern of these vessels shown in 24G indicates that they are dilated normal vessels rather than a vascular malformation; and there is certainly no evidence of enlarged feeding or draining vessels. Patchy contrast enhancement seen in the infarct may be seen from the end of the first week to as long as six months and is a feature of subacute infarction. The diagnosis was confirmed angiographically (24I) where the arrow points to the occluded right middle cerebral artery.

Reference

1. Bradley WG. Ischemia. In: Bradley WG, Bydder G. *MRI atlas of the brain.* London: Martin Dunitz, 1990;143–181.

Submitted by: Stephen J. Davis, M.D. and Louis M. Teresi, M.D., Huntington Medical Research Institutes, Pasadena, California; William G. Bradley, Jr., M.D., Ph.D., Senior Editor.

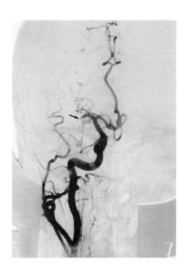

FIG. 24I. Angiogram.

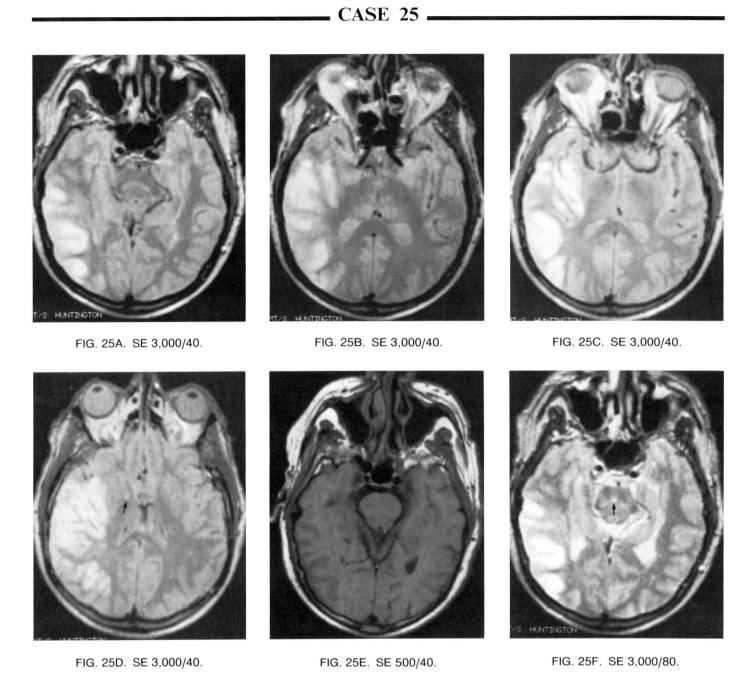

FIG. 25A. SE 3,000/40.   FIG. 25B. SE 3,000/40.   FIG. 25C. SE 3,000/40.

FIG. 25D. SE 3,000/40.   FIG. 25E. SE 500/40.   FIG. 25F. SE 3,000/80.

Clinical History

A 65-year-old male with sudden onset of left-sided weakness, numbness, and slurring of speech 24 hours prior to MRI.

Findings

Axial 5 mm T2-W (SE 3,000/40 and 80) images are presented.

There is a large area of cortically based high signal on the T2-weighted sequences involving the lateral aspect of the right temporal and inferior right parietal lobes with involvement of the underlying insular cortex (25A–25D). On the T1-weighted sequence, this region shows decreased signal intensity in a gyriform pattern with mild cerebral swelling as evidenced by effacement of the local cortical sulci (25E). There is a normal flow void within the visualized proximal middle cerebral arterial circulation and there is no MR evidence of hemorrhage.

Mucoperiosteal thickening is present in the ethmoid and left frontal sinuses. There is a 3 mm lacune inferiorly in the right anterior limb of the internal capsule (25D, arrow) and scattered foci of high signal are also noted in the deep white matter, consistent with deep white matter ischemia or infarction.

A 5 mm diameter focus of high signal in the central pons (25F, arrow), represents partial volume effect of the CSF in the inferior aspect of the interpeduncular cistern. As there is no evidence of this on the first echo (25A), this should not be confused with a brainstem infarct.

Diagnosis

Acute infarction in the distribution of the right middle cerebral artery.

Discussion

In the acute phase, MR imaging is more sensitive than CT scanning in the depiction of cerebral infarction due to its increased sensitivity to elevation of tissue water. MR imaging depicts virtually all infarcts over the age of six hours, whereas CT shows, at best, 75% of infarcts at 24 hours. The increase in free water content is due to breakdown of cellular membrane pumps. However, the overall increase in water content and, therefore, mass effect is small in the acute infarct. Prolongation of the T1 and T2 relaxation times is caused in the early stages of ischemia by intracellular water accumulation. As the infarct evolves and vasogenic edema begins to accumulate, accompanying proteins cause a relative decrease in the prolongation of the T1 and T2 relaxation values due to hydration layer water effects. This patient had a normal CT scan performed 12 hours prior to this study.

Reference

1. Brant-Zawadzki M. Ischemia. In: Stark DD, Bradley WG, eds. *Magnetic resonance imaging.* St. Louis: C.V. Mosby Co., 1988;299–315.

Submitted by: Stephen J. Davis, M.D. and Louis M. Teresi, M.D., Huntington Medical Research Institutes, Pasadena, California; William G. Bradley, Jr., M.D., Ph.D., Senior Editor.

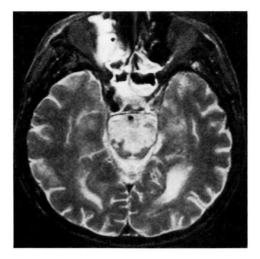

FIG. 26A. SE 2,800/90.

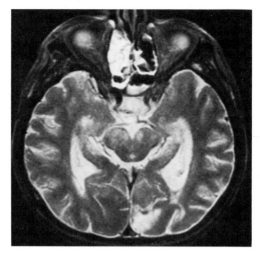

FIG. 26B. SE 2,800/90.

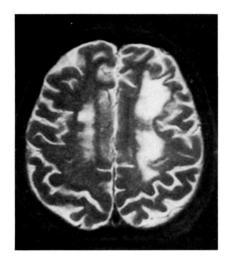

FIG. 26C. SE 2,800/90.

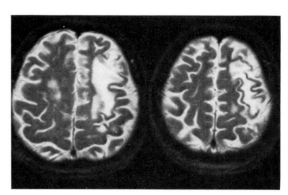

FIG. 26D. SE 2,800/90.

Clinical History

A 69-year-old male with sudden onset of paralysis, five days prior to MRI. Now comatose, on respirator.

Findings

The series of T2-weighted axial images (26A–26D) documents an extensive area of edematous infarction in the pons. Note the higher sections show evidence of similar abnormality in the left occipital pole (26B), as well as in the watershed/border zone between the posterior cerebral and middle cerebral, as well as the anterior cerebral and middle cerebral territories of the left hemisphere (26C, 26D).

Closer attention to the lowest cut (26A) reveals absence of the normal signal void within the left internal carotid artery, although some reconstitution is seen at the level of the optic foramen (26B), most likely due to an ophthalmic retrograde pathway. Note the basilar artery shows normal signal void (26A).

Diagnosis

A large pontine infarct as well as watershed infarction of the left hemisphere.

Discussion

Pontine infarcts of this size generally result from an embolic episode into the basilar artery distribution. Symmetric bilateral pontine infarction generally appears due to ischemia in the distribution of the multiple perforating arteries off the basilar that feed the pons. The clot often fragments after several days and may migrate distally. Posterior cerebral territory may be at risk as well.

Of interest in this case is the rather limited infarction of the left hemisphere given the combination of posterior circulation insult and left internal carotid artery occlusion. Note that the major anterior cerebral and middle cerebral artery territories remain perfused, but, at the periphery of the territories (the "watershed"), ischemia did develop due to hypoperfusion. This watershed territory is nicely delineated by the upper slices on this study.

References

1. Brant-Zawadzki M et al. MR imaging and spectroscopy in clinical and experimental cerebral ischemia: a review. *AJNR* 1987;8:39–48.
2. Sipponen J et al. Serial nuclear magnetic resonance imaging in patients with cerebral infarction. *J Comput Assist Tomogr* 1983;7:585–589.
3. Kistler J et al. Vertebral basilar posterior cerebral territory stroke—delineation by proton nuclear magnetic resonance imaging. *Stroke* 1984;15:417–426.

Submitted by: Roger Bird, M.D., Barrow Neurologic Institute, Phoenix, Arizona; Michael Brant-Zawadzki, M.D., Senior Editor.

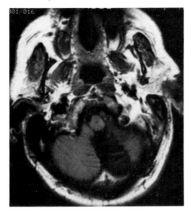

FIG. 27A. SE 800/20.

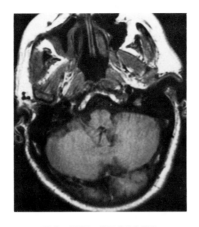

FIG. 27B. SE 800/20.

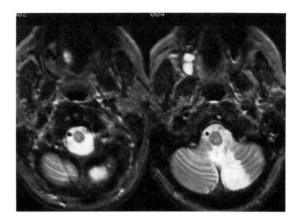

FIG. 27C. SE 2,800/90.

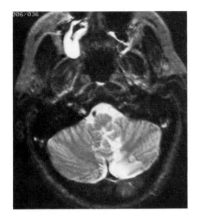

FIG. 27D. SE 2,800/90.

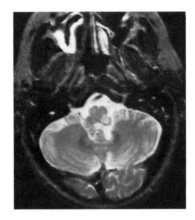

FIG. 27E. SE 2,800/90.

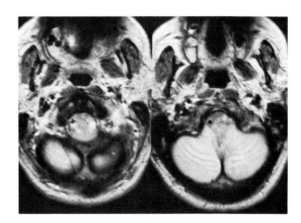

FIG. 27F. SE 2,800/30.

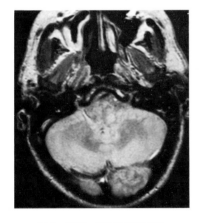

FIG. 27G. SE 2,800/30.

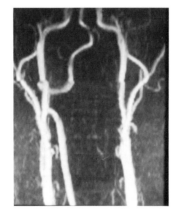

FIG. 27H. MR angiogram.

Clinical History

A 61-year-old male with dysphagia, hoarseness, vertigo, nystagmus, left facial numbness, and altered sensation, right side of body—sudden onset four months prior to the current study.

Findings

The T1-weighted axial images in the posterior fossa reveal an irregular, roughly oval area of low signal intensity in the inferior aspect of the left cerebellar hemisphere (27A, 27B). The T2-weighted second echo images show a corresponding abnormality with high signal intensity in this distribution (27C–27E), as well as showing a focal 1 cm lesion in the left dorsal-lateral medulla. Of interest, the first echo images show relatively little abnormality on corresponding sections (27F, 27G). Careful scrutiny of the two vertebral arteries on the axial cuts reveals a normal appearance of the right vertebral artery but high signal within the left vertebral artery, which also appears hypoplastic. The MR angiogram verifies a single, large right vertebral, with only a small remnant of the left vertebral shown just below the vertebral basilar junction (27H).

Diagnosis

Posterior-inferior cerebral artery (PICA) infarction; left vertebral occlusive disease.

Discussion

The abnormality here is in the typical distribution of the posterior-inferior cerebral artery and has the classic appearance of a remote infarction. The low signal intensity on the T1-weighted sequences matches that of normal CSF, and the impression is verified on the first and second echo sequences. Bulk water has replaced normal brain substance (macrocystic encephalomalacia) in the inferior cerebellar hemispheres supplied by the PICA. Note that the smaller lesion of the medulla does not contain bulk water, rather the picture is that of microcystic encephalomalacia—that is, loose tissue with increased extra cellular water that produces a relatively higher signal on the first echo of the T2-weighted sequence (due to the T1-shortening effect of the proteinaceous tissue) than would a bulk water collection. The absence of mass effect, in fact, evidence of loss of brain substance, indicates this to be an insult of greater than three to four weeks' duration. Cerebral infarction will show mass effect for the first two to three weeks if large enough, due to the vasogenic edema component, but it will eventually lead to local atrophy (starting three to four weeks after the insult).

Finally, the observation of a small left vertebral artery that contains signal within it is further proof of ischemia as the cause of the lesion. The MR angiogram verifies this impression.

The clinical description in the history is classic for the lateral medullary syndrome of Wallenberg. The vertigo, nausea, and vomiting result from involvement of the vestibular nuclei; the facial analgesia is caused by involvement of the descending tract and nucleus of the 5th nerve. Loss of normal sensation in the contralateral part of the body results from involvement of the spinothalamic tract. All these structures can be found in the distribution of the PICA.

References

1. Brant-Zawadzki M et al. MR imaging and spectroscopy in clinical and experimental cerebral ischemia: a review. *AJNR* 1987;8:39–48.
2. Sipponen J et al. Serial nuclear magnetic resonance imaging in patients with cerebral infarction. *J Comput Assist Tomogr* 1983;7:585–589.
3. Kistler J et al. Vertebral basilar posterior cerebral territory stroke—delineation by proton nuclear magnetic resonance imaging. *Stroke* 1984;15:417–426.
4. Duncan G et al. Acute cerebellar infarction in the PICA territory. *Arch Neurol* 1975;32:364–368.

Submitted by: Roger Bird, M.D., Barrow Neurologic Institute, Phoenix, Arizona; Michael Brant-Zawadzki, M.D., Senior Editor.

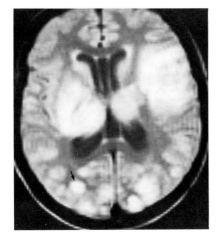

FIG. 28A. SE 2,000/30.

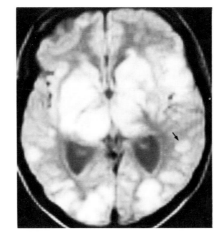

FIG. 28B. SE 2,000/30.

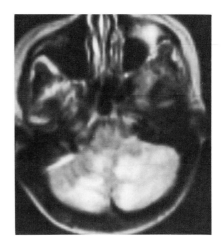

FIG. 28C. SE 2,000/60.

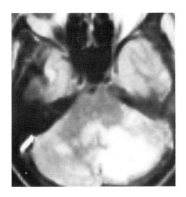

FIG. 28D. SE 2,000/60.

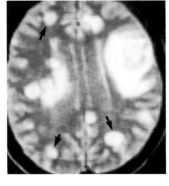

FIG. 28E. SE 2,000/60.

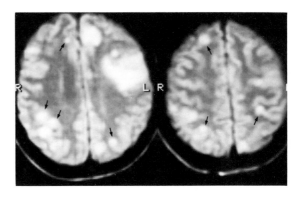

FIG. 28F. SE 2,000/30.

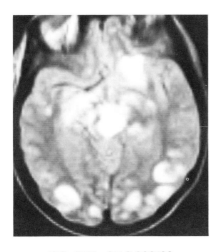

FIG. 28G. SE 2,000/60.

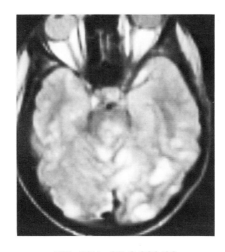

FIG. 28H. SE 2,000/60.

Clinical History

A 32-year-old female with five-year history of nephritis presents with sudden blindness in the right eye and acute onset of depression, mutism, memory problems, progressive weakness, and inability to walk. She is taking high-dose Prednisolone for her nephritis. Examination revealed bilateral retinal vasculitis, right 3rd nerve palsy, and a peripheral sensory neuropathy.

60

Findings

Axial 10 mm T2-W (SE 2,000/30 and 60) images are presented.

There are diffuse focal parenchymal lesions involving both the supra- and infra-tentorial compartments. Several lesions are cortically-based, including a 6 cm lesion involving the left posterior frontal lobe (28A), several 2–3 cm lesions involving both occipital and posterior parietal lobes (28A, 28B), and bilateral cortically based cerebellar lesions (28C, 28D). In addition to these cortically based lesions, there are multiple 1–2 cm diameter lesions involving the white matter, predominantly centered at the gray-white junction (28A, 28B, 28E, 28F, black arrows). There are large confluent lesions involving the basal ganglia bilaterally, more marked on the right side (28A, 28B), with bilateral thalamic lesions ex-tending to involve the upper midbrain (28G, 28H). In addition to the bilateral, cortically-based cerebellar lesions, there are lesions in the deep white matter of the cerebellum bilaterally, more marked on the left side (28C, 28D).

There is mass effect involving the bilateral thalamic, basal ganglia, midbrain, and bilateral cerebellar lesions, resulting in mild ventricular obstruction at the level of the cerebral aqueduct, evidenced by dilatation of the lateral ventricles and a thin, smooth rim of periventricular high signal intensity indicating obstructive hydrocephalus (28A, 28B, 28E). A cavum septum pellucidum (28A) and vergae (28E) are noted. There is no MR evidence of hemorrhage.

Diagnosis

Extensive cerebral vasculitis secondary to systemic lupus erythematosis (SLE) with multiple vasculitic infarcts; mild acute obstructive hydrocephalus.

Discussion

Cerebral arteritis may involve the large arteries at the base of the brain, the convexity branches, or the smaller intracerebral arterioles. The arteritis associated with SLE involves predominantly the small cerebral arteries. This change results in small infarcts involving the cortex and subcortical regions. Small arteries supplying the basal ganglia and internal capsules are also involved, as in this case. Arteritic involvement of the large arteries at the base of the brain and the medium-sized arteries of the cerebral cortex also occurs and causes more typical cerebral hemispheric infarcts. In this case, arteritis of the thalamoperforating branches of the posterior cerebral artery causes extensive acute infarction of the thalami and upper midbrain. The mass effect of these infarcts leads to aqueductal obstruction and hydrocephalus.

Lupus vasculitis characteristically involves the cortex in addition to the subcortical white matter, and it is this peripheral distribution that helps differentiate it from other causes of predominantly white matter disease, such as multiple sclerosis. Many of the lesions may resolve following steroid therapy, indicating that some may involve ischemic, cytotoxic edema rather than the vasogenic edema that follows infarction. Other causes of primary cerebral arteritis include giant cell arteritis, sarcoidosis, granulomatous arteritis, and chemical arteritis secondary to intravenous amphetamine, cocaine, or heroine abuse. Arteritis also arises secondary to cerebral infective inflammatory diseases.

In patients on high-dose steroids, opportunistic infections such as toxoplasmosis would also need to be considered, although the distribution in this case, with both cortically and subcortically based lesions, strongly favors vasculitis as an etiology. The clinical finding of retinal vasculitis is strong supporting evidence.

References

1. Miller DH, Ormerod IEC, Gibson A, et al. MR brain scanning in patients with vasculitis: differentiation from multiple sclerosis. *Neuroradiology* 1987;29:226.
2. Aisen AM, Gabrielsen TO, McCune WJ. MR imaging of systemic lupus erythematosis involving the brain. *AJNR* 1985;6:197–202.

Submitted by: Stephen J. Davis, M.D. and Louis M. Teresi, M.D., Huntington Medical Research Institutes, Pasadena, California; William G. Bradley, Jr., M.D., Ph.D., Senior Editor.

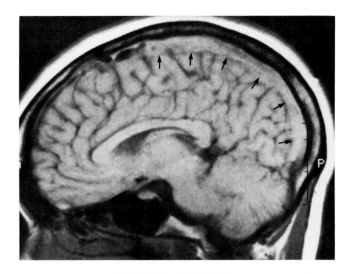

FIG. 29A. SE 500/30.

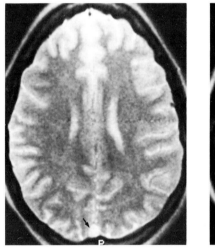

FIG. 29B. SE 3,000/80.

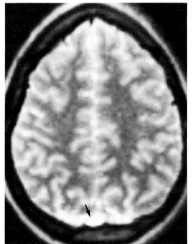

FIG. 29C. SE 3,000/80.

Clinical History

A 20-year-old female with recent onset of headaches.

Findings

Axial 5 mm T2-W (SE 3,000/80) and sagittal 10 mm T1-W (SE 500/30) images are presented.

The normal flow void of the superior sagittal sinus is replaced by increased signal intensity tissue on both the sagittal T1-weighted images (29A, black arrows) and axial T2-weighted images (29B, 29C, black arrows). The flow void is lost throughout the posterior two-thirds of the sagittal sinus as far posteriorly as its junction with the straight sinus, where a normal flow void is again seen. There is no evidence of cortical infarction, hemorrhagic infarction, or undue distention of the cortical veins.

Diagnosis

Sagittal sinus thrombosis without evidence of venous infarction.

Discussion

Cerebral veno-occlusive disease may be caused by adjacent infective processes, tumors (particularly meningiomas and leukemia), regional trauma (particularly with fractures extending into the dural sinus), and low flow and hypercoagulable states. Other associated disorders include dehydration, post-operative states, and diabetes mellitus with ketoacidosis. Patients may present with a wide spectrum of disorders from a relatively mild headache to severe disorders including paresis, convulsions, and raised intracranial pressure.

Venous occlusion has also been related to benign intracranial hypertension, a condition more common in young women. This may relate to the association of veno-occlusive disease with menstrual dysfunction, pregnancy, and oral contraceptive pills. Veno-occlusive disease is likely to be underdiagnosed, which is particularly unfortunate as the prognosis is directly related to the rapidity with which treatment is instituted.

In this patient, the sagittal sinus is filled with thrombus. While this condition may be associated with dilated cortical veins, hemorrhagic venous infarction, and cerebral edema, none of these is present in this case. Difficulties in diagnosing venous sinus occlusion on MR include the differentiation of flow-related enhancement and slow flow from intraluminal clot.

These may be distinguished by visualizing the suspected thrombus in multiple planes or by the use of single-slice gradient echo acquisitions or phase imaging techniques, both of which are sensitive to flow. Presaturation pulses can be used to eliminate flow-related enhancement.

Reference

1. Sze G, Simmons B, Kroll G, et al. Dural sinus thrombosis: verification with spin echo techniques. *AJNR* 1988;9:679–686.

Submitted by: Stephen J. Davis, M.D. and Louis M. Teresi, M.D., Huntington Medical Research Institutes, Pasadena, California; William G. Bradley, M.D., Ph.D., Senior Editor.

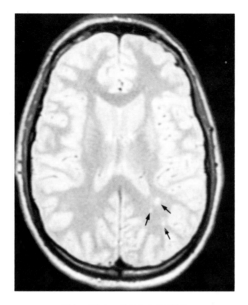

FIG. 30A. SE 3,000/40.

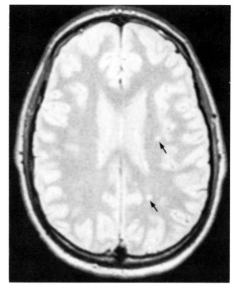

FIG. 30B. SE 3,000/40.

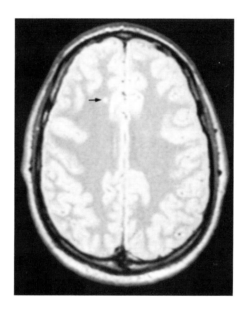

FIG. 30C. SE 3,000/40.

Clinical History

An 18-year-old male with multiple episodes of severe headaches intermittently for 18 months.

Findings

Axial 5 mm mildly T2-W (SE 3,000/40) images are presented.

There are scattered punctate foci measuring 2–5 mm in diameter scattered throughout the periventricular white matter and in the centrum semiovale with some prominence about the left periatrial region (30A–30C, black arrows).

Diagnosis

Migraine-related deep white matter abnormality.

Discussion

Focal deep white matter abnormalities have been noted in patients with classic migraine. These patients need not have a history of a complicated or hemiplegic migraine and do not have neurological deficits. Although the nature of these lesions has not yet been established, they may be due to small deep white matter infarcts secondary to vascular spasm associated with migraine. Complicated migraine is associated with neurological deficits that are usually transient. In addition, cortical abnormalities (probably infarcts) have been documented; these lesions are not seen in patients with uncomplicated migraine.

The differential diagnosis includes multiple sclerosis. A periatrial distribution of lesions, brainstem or posterior fossa lesions, and a history of multiple episodes of recurrent neurological deficit would favor this diagnosis. This patient had no clinical or CSF evidence to support multiple sclerosis. A vasculitis involving the small arterioles seen, for example, in connective tissue diseases or with intravenous drug abuse could also present similar appearances. Evidence of cortical infarcts or basal ganglia infarcts and a relevant clinical history would help to favor the diagnosis of arteritis. These are the predominant differential diagnoses in patients under the age of 50. In patients over the age of 50, deep white matter infarction often associated with hypertension or diabetes, but also often seen in the absence of these diseases, becomes increasingly common, with 60% of patients over the age of 60 years showing some periventricular white-matter abnormality.

References

1. Soges LJ, Cacayorin ED, Ramuchandron TS, et al. Migraine: evaluation by MRI. *AJNR* 1988;9:45–49.
2. Bradley WG, Whittemore AR, Watanabe AS, Homyok M, Teresi LM, Davis SJ. Association of deep white matter infarction with chronic communicating hydrocephalus: implications regarding the possible etiology of normal pressure hydrocephalus. *AJNR*. (In press.)

Submitted by: Stephen J. Davis, M.D. and Louis M. Teresi, M.D., Huntington Medical Research Institutes, Pasadena, California; William G. Bradley, M.D., Ph.D., Senior Editor.

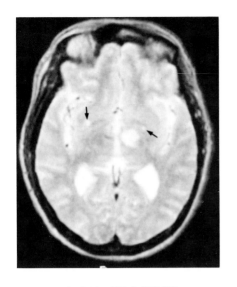

FIG. 31A. SE 3,000/80.

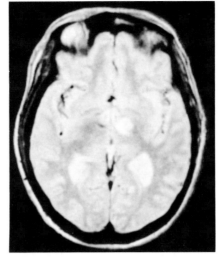

FIG. 31B. SE 3,000/40.

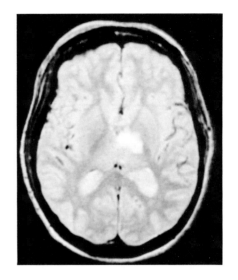

FIG. 31C. SE 3,000/40.

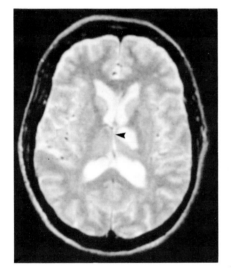

FIG. 31D. SE 3,000/80.

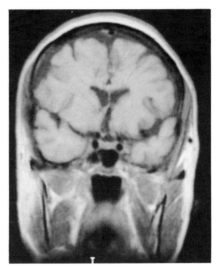

FIG. 31E. SE 500/30.

Clinical History

A 70-year-old woman presents with sudden onset of slurred of speech and altered cognition three days prior to the scan; profound recent memory loss.

Findings

Axial 5 mm T2-W (SE 3,000/40 and 80) and coronal 10 mm T1-W (SE 500/30) images are presented.

There is a 1.5 × 2.0 cm lesion involving the anterior aspect of the left thalamus extending into the adjacent posterior rim of the internal capsule (31A–31D). This is causing mild mass effect with displacement of the 3rd ventricle toward the right (31D, arrowhead). There is no evidence of ventricular obstruction. There is no alteration in the signal intensity in this region on the T1-weighted sequence (31E).

Two high-intensity punctate foci are seen related to the anterior commissure: one anterior to the right anterior commissure and one just posterior to the left anterior commissure (31A, arrows). These are seen only on the most T2-weighted sequence and are not visualized on the first echo of the long TR sequence, indicating that their intensity follows that of CSF in dilated perivascular space.

Diagnosis

Acute thalamic infarct; dilated perivascular spaces.

Discussion

Lacunes are small cavities with a diameter of less than 1 cm and are the result of small deep infarcts due to thrombotic occlusion of individual penetrating arteries, typically involving the internal capsule or basal ganglia. The next most frequent site is in the basis pontis. They typically spare the cerebral and cerebellar cortex. Histologically, hemosiderin-laden macrophages often occur around the cavity suggesting that small hemorrhages are also common, although it is not common to see evidence of this at MR. Systemic hypertension is associated in over 90% of cases, and there is a frequent (35%) association of putaminal and thalamic hemorrhage with lacunar disease. Clinically, they result in abrupt neurological deficit without a change in state of consciousness, recovery from which is often significant.

The thalamus is supplied by thalamoperforating branches of the posterior cerebral artery. Thalamic infarcts may cause personality change and memory loss (as in this case), extrapyramidal-type motor syndromes, mental arousal, dysphagia, and pain syndromes. This lesion has mass effect that is prominent for an infarct three days following its onset. Mass effect from acute infarction increases over the first week and usually begins to resolve by the third week. In chronic lacunes, T1-weighted images are useful, as they show decreased signal intensity due to the small cavitations present. In addition, their typical position and evidence of any adjacent hemorrhage helps to differentiate these lesions from other processes such as demyelinating disease.

Perivascular spaces are common in the inferior basal ganglia adjacent to the anterior commissure.

Reference

1. Fisher CM. Lacunar strokes and infarcts: a review. *Neurology* 1982;32:871–876.

Submitted by: Stephen J. Davis, M.D. and Louis M. Teresi, M.D., Huntington Medical Research Institutes, Pasadena, California; William G. Bradley, Jr., M.D., Ph.D., Senior Editor.

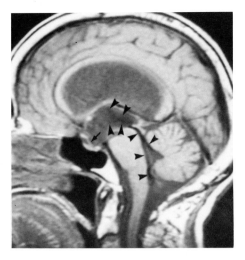

FIG. 32A. SE 500/20.

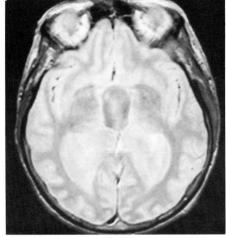

FIG. 32B. SE 3,000/30.

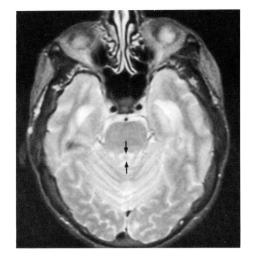

FIG. 32C. SE 3,000/70.

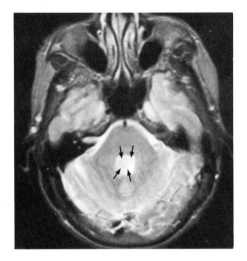

FIG. 32D. SE 3,000/70.

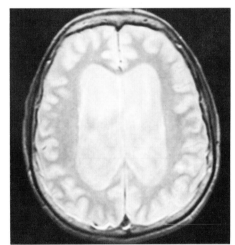

FIG. 32E. SE 3,000/30.

Clinical History

A 61-year-old woman with ataxia and memory impairment.

Findings

Axial 5 mm T2-W (SE 3,000/30 and 70) and sagittal 5 mm T1-W (SE 500/20) images are presented.

There is marked symmetrical dilatation of the ventricular system, particularly involving the 3rd and lateral ventricles (32A, 32B, 32E). Of note is dilatation of the chiasmatic and infundibular recesses of the 3rd ventricle with forward displacement of the pituitary stalk (32A, black arrow). There is no accompanying dilatation of the cerebral sulci or basal cisterns, and there is upward bowing of the corpus callosum and flattening of the cortical gyri against the inner table of the calvarium, best seen on the sagittal view (32A). There is a very prominent CSF flow void (32A, arrowheads) through a dilated cerebral aqueduct extending along the 4th ventricle to the level of the obex and along the superior roof of the 4th ventricle adjacent to the superior medullary velum. This indicates both patency of the cerebral aqueduct and a hyperdynamic CSF flow state. The aqueduct is dilated. Signal loss due to turbulence from hyperdynamic retrograde CSF flow can be seen occupying most of the 3rd ventricle (32B). The flow void is also seen throughout the length of the 4th ventricle on the sagittal images (32A, arrow).

Diagnosis

Normal pressure hydrocephalus (NPH).

Discussion

Communicating hydrocephalus is distinguished from atrophy by the disproportionate enlargement of the ventricular system compared to the cortical sulci. The findings here are typical with marked dilatation of the ventricular system, upward bowing of the corpus callosum, flattening of the gyri against the inner table of the skull, and a prominent CSF flow void through the cerebral aqueduct. The CSF flow void is due to turbulent dephasing of the water protons produced by increased velocity. These dephased protons result in reduced signal intensity.

One form of chronic communicating hydrocephalus is so-called *normal pressure hydrocephalus*, where elderly patients present with gait apraxia followed by memory loss and incontinence. Because some of these patients will respond to ventricular shunting, the identification of these cases is clinically important. However, the diagnosis has been controversial, and no reliable criteria have been clearly established. A recent study has shown the *extent* of the CSF flow void to be related to the surgical outcome, i.e., patients with an extensive flow void were most likely to respond to ventricular shunting. These patients had a flow void that extended throughout the length of the 4th ventricle due to hyperdynamic, antegrade CSF flow during cardiac systole. A similar flow void due to retrograde diastolic flow extended into the 3rd ventricle and occasionally back into the lateral ventricles via the foramen of Monro.

Reference

1. Bradley WG, Whittemore AR, Watanabe AS, Homyak M, Teresi LM, Davis SJ. Marked CSF flow void: an indicator of successful shunting in patients with suspected normal pressure hydrocephalus. *Radiology*. (In press).

Submitted by: Stephen J. Davis, M.D. and Louis M. Teresi, M.D., Huntington Medical Research Institutes, Pasadena, California; William G. Bradley, Jr., M.D., Ph.D., Senior Editor.

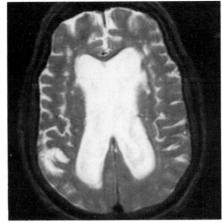

FIG. 33A. SE 2,800/80.

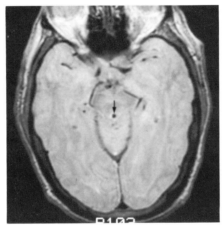

FIG. 33B. SE 2,800/80.

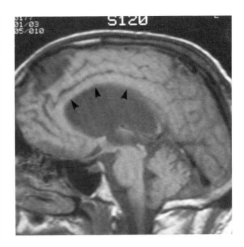

FIG. 33C. SE 500/20.

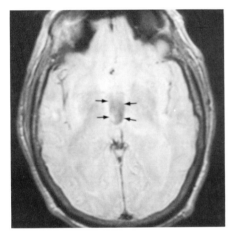

FIG. 33D. SE 2,800/30.

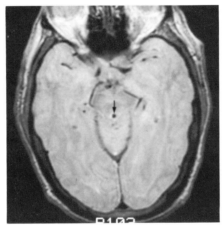

FIG. 33E. SE 2,800/30.

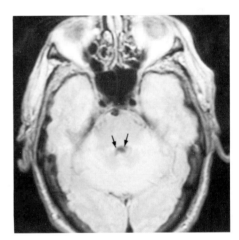

FIG. 33F. SE 2,800/30.

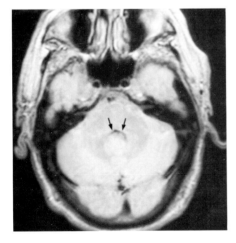

FIG. 33G. SE 2,800/30.

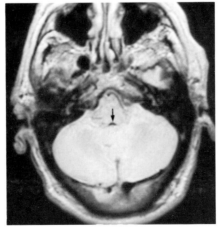

FIG. 33H. SE 2,800/30.

Clinical History

A 75-year-old man with progressive ataxia and recent memory loss.

Findings

Axial 5 mm T2-W (SE 2,800/30 and 80) and sagittal 5 mm T1-W (SE 500/20) are presented.

There is prominent dilatation of the lateral and 3rd ventricles (33A, 33B). On the saggital view, there is upward bowing of the corpus callosum (33C, arrowheads) and flattening of the cortical gyri. There is an extensive CSF flow void extending from the 3rd ventricle (33D) through the cerebral aqueduct (33E) into the 4th ventricle (33F, 33H, black arrows) with marked signal loss in the aqueduct. The flow void extends cranially back through the 3rd ventricle to the level of the foramen of Monro (33A, 33D, arrows) and caudally along the floor of the 4th ventricle to the level of the obex (33H, arrow).

There is mild prominence of the cortical sulci in the frontal regions consistent with cortical atrophy. Multiple punctate and confluent areas of increased signal intensity are present in the periventricular white matter bilaterally (33B).

Diagnosis

1. Communicating hydrocephalus with hyperdynamic CSF flow: normal pressure hydrocephalus (NPH).
2. Periventricular deep white matter ischemic changes.

Discussion

This patient has classical features of communicating hydrocephalus and a clinical presentation typical of normal pressure hydrocephalus. The features of this condition are discussed in Case 32.

Widespread periventricular hyperintensities are also more common in these patients than in the normal population, and the two processes are statistically related. A recent study shows that chronic communicating hydrocephalus with increased CSF flow void is statistically related to deep white matter infarction and that the presence of deep white matter infarction should not be considered a contraindication to ventriculo-peritoneal shunting in patients with suspected normal pressure hydrocephalus. However, the association of these two disorders is not invariable. Other causes of communicating hydrocephalus include meningeal inflammatory or neoplastic processes and subarachnoid hemorrhage.

Reference

1. Bradley WG, Whittemore AR, Watanabe AS, Homyak M, Davis SJ, Teresi LM. Association of deep white matter infarction with chronic communicating hydrocephalus: implications regarding the possible etiology of normal pressure hydrocephalus. *AJNR*. (In press).

Submitted by: Stephen J. Davis, M.D. and Louis M. Teresi, M.D., Huntington Medical Research Institutes, Pasadena, California; William G. Bradley, Jr., M.D., Ph.D., Senior Editor.

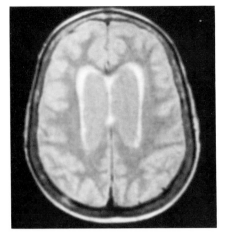

FIG. 34A. SE 3,000/40.

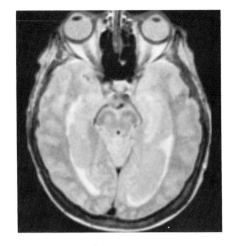

FIG. 34B. SE 3,000/40.

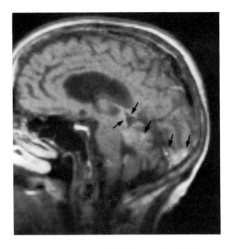

FIG. 34C. SE 500/40 with Gd-DTPA.

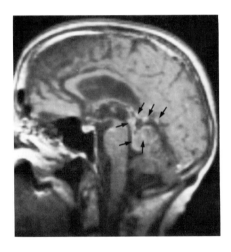

FIG. 34D. SE 500/40 with Gd-DTPA.

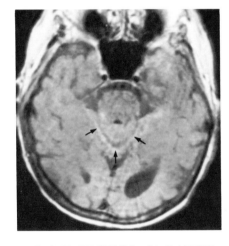

FIG. 34E. SE 750/30 with Gd-DTPA.

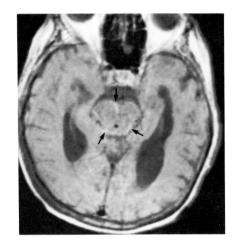

FIG. 34F. SE 750/30 with Gd-DTPA.

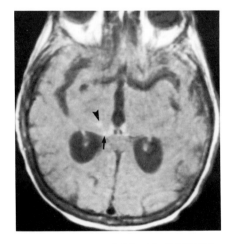

FIG. 34G. SE 750/30 with Gd-DTPA.

Clinical History

A 76-year-old woman with carcinoma of the lung and seven days of headaches and confusion.

Findings

Axial 5 mm T2-W (SE 3,000/40) and axial and sagittal gadolinium-enhanced 5 mm T1-W (SE 500–750/40) images are presented.

The ventricles are moderately enlarged, and the lateral ventricles are surrounded by a smooth rim of increased signal intensity on the T2-weighted images (34A, 34B). There is a normal (but not increased) flow void through the aqueduct. In addition to the smooth periventricular border, there is also a patchy component secondary to mild, deep white matter ischemia.

Mucosal thickening is noted in the paranasal sinuses.

After gadolinium diethylenetriamine penta-acetic acid (DTPA) administration, there is meningeal enhancement noted surrounding the pontine isthmus, midbrain, quadrigeminal plate cistern, and superior vermian cistern (34C–34G, arrows). There is also minimal enhancement of the sylvian cisterns bilaterally. There is a 3 mm enhancing nodule posteriorly in the right thalamus (34G, arrowhead).

Diagnosis

Acute communicating hydrocephalus secondary to leptomeningeal metastatic disease; thalamic metastatic nodule.

Discussion

The smooth rim of periventricular increased signal on the T2-weighted images is typical of interstitial edema from transependymal resorption of CSF. As the intraventricular pressure rises, a smooth periventricular border is rapidly formed. If the obstruction persists for a few weeks, the interstitial edema leaches out lipid in the myelin and increases the relative water content of the periventricular tissues. Thus, the smooth border of high intensity does not resolve immediately after shunting until remyelination occurs. In chronic obstruction, the ventricles continue to dilate and the pressure decreases to near-normal levels, eventually with loss of the smooth periventricular border. The hydrocephalus is then said to be *compensated*. Smooth periventricular increased intensity can also be caused by central tracking of vasogenic edema (of any cause) produced in the cerebral hemispheres.

Communicating hydrocephalus may be due to obstruction in the basal cisterns from carcinomatous or infectious meningitis. Similarly, obstruction of the arachnoid villi may be caused by these processes or by subarachnoid hemorrhage. Carcinomatous meningitis is often caused by an extracranial malignancy such as carcinoma of the breast, lung, or lymphoma. Subarachnoid spread of intra-axial lesions such as medulloblastoma, primitive neuroectodermal tumor (PNET) or ependymoma is more common in children. Cortical venous thrombosis or sagittal sinus thrombosis may also cause communicating hydrocephalus.

Reference

1. Bradley WG Jr. Hydrocephalus and atrophy. In: Stark DD, Bradley WG, eds. *Magnetic resonance imaging*, Chapt. 22. St. Louis: C.V. Mosby Co., 1988.

Submitted by: Stephen J. Davis, M.D. and Louis M. Teresi, M.D., Huntington Medical Research Institutes, Pasadena, California; William G. Bradley, Jr., M.D., Ph.D., Senior Editor.

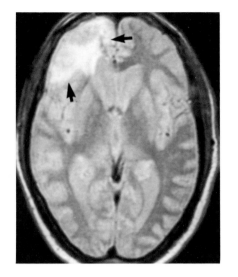

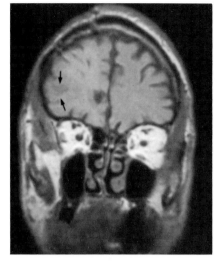

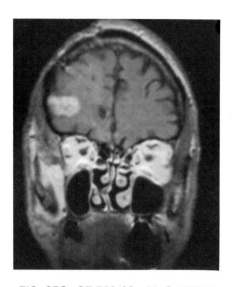

FIG. 35A. SE 3,000/40.　　　　FIG. 35B. SE 750/30.　　　　FIG. 35C. SE 750/30 with Gd-DTPA.

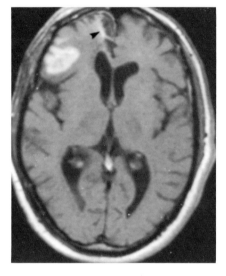

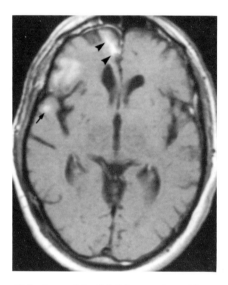

FIG. 35D. SE 500/30 with Gd-DTPA.　　　FIG. 35E. SE 500/30 with Gd-DTPA.

Clinical History

A 59-year-old male with previous history of resected right frontal lobe metastasis and subsequent radiation therapy 18 months previously.

Findings

Axial 5 mm T2-W (SE 3,000/40), and coronal pre-gadolinium and coronal and axial post-gadolinium T1-W (SE 500–750/30) images are presented.

There is a cortically based wedge-shaped area of increased signal intensity on the T2-weighted sequence (35A, black arrows) in the anterior right frontal lobe. The lesion predominantly involves the white matter but also involves the overlying cortex. There is an ill-defined, rounded 1.5 cm mass lesion shown in this region on the pre-gadolinium T1-weighted sequence (35B, black arrows) that shows evidence of mass effect with effacement of the overlying cortical sulci. Following gadolinium administration, this region shows a thick 5 mm to 1 cm rind of contrast enhancement (35C, 35D). A further 5 mm nodule of enhancement is shown in the right temporal operculum (35E, black arrow). Irregular enhancement is present in the margins of the defect residual from the previous surgery (35D, 35E, arrowheads). Evidence of the previous right frontal craniotomy is noted.

A second set of 5 mm gadolinium-enhanced T1-W (SE 750/30) images taken following excision of the two described lesions is also presented. These show evidence of excisional biopsy of the right temporal opercular lesion (35F) and the right frontal lesion (35G).

Diagnosis

Post-irradiation necrosis producing mass effect and simulating tumor recurrence.

Discussion

Both of these lesions would be typical of malignancy, with the right temporal operculum nodule situated at the gray-white interface (typical of metastatic disease) and the right frontal lesion showing irregular ring contrast enhancement and focal mass effect. However, both of these lesions were proved to be due to radiation necrosis only by histological analysis. Radiation injury produces thickening and hyalinization of the arteriolar wall and subsequent parenchymal necrosis. Parenchymal necrosis has a latent period of one month to 14 years and generally occurs with doses of 6,000 rad or greater. Radiation necrosis may appear as an irregular region of enhancement without mass effect, as a solitary area of enhancement with or without mass effect, or, as in this case, as a ring lesion simulating recurrent tumor or abscess. Differentiation can be made only by biopsy or long-term follow up.

Reference

1. Curnes JT, Laster DW, Ball MR. Magnetic resonance imaging of radiation injury to the brain. *AJNR* 1986;7:389–394.

Submitted by: Stephen J. Davis, M.D. and Louis M. Teresi, M.D., Huntington Medical Research Institutes, Pasadena, California; William G. Bradley, Jr., M.D., Ph.D., Senior Editor.

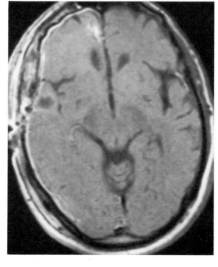

FIG. 35F. SE 750/30 with Gd-DTPA.

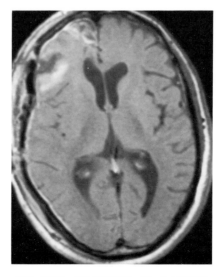

FIG. 35G. SE 750/30 with Gd-DTPA.

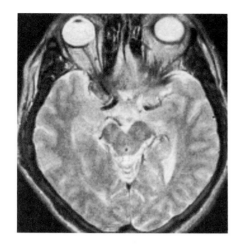

FIG. 36A. SE 3,000/80.

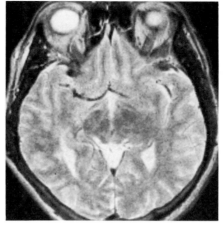

FIG. 36B. SE 3,000/80.

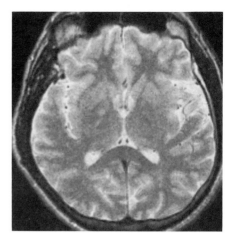

FIG. 36C. SE 3,000/80.

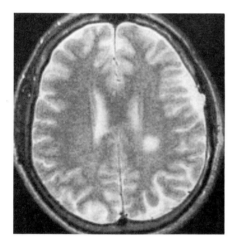

FIG. 36D. SE 3,000/80.

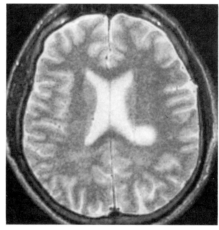

FIG. 36E. SE 3,000/80.

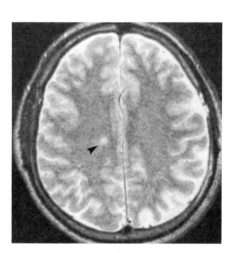

FIG. 36F. SE 3,000/80.

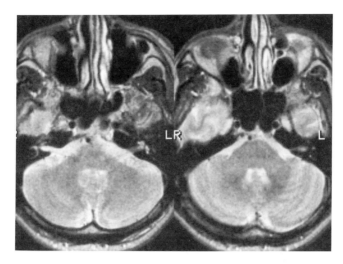

FIG. 36G. SE 3,000/80.

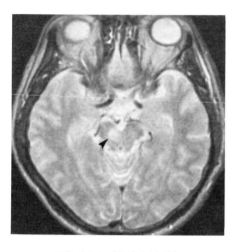

FIG. 36H. SE 3,000/80.

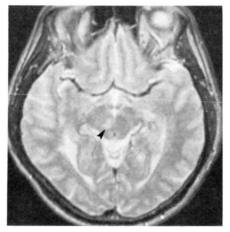

FIG. 36I. SE 3,000/80.

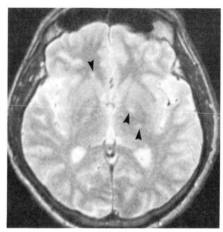

FIG. 36J. SE 3,000/80.

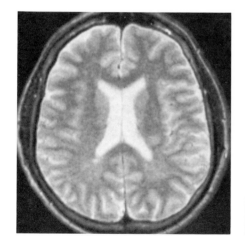

FIG. 36K. SE 3,000/80.

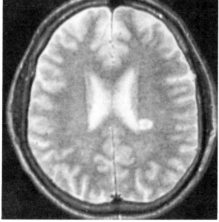

FIG. 36L. SE 3,000/80.

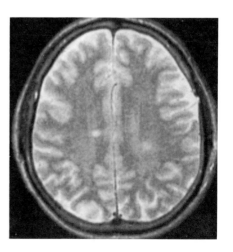

FIG. 36M. SE 3,000/80.

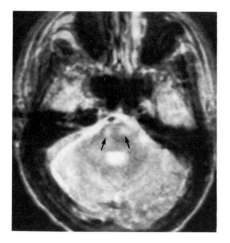

FIG. 36N. SE 3,000/80.

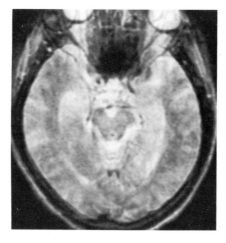

FIG. 36O. SE 3,000/80.

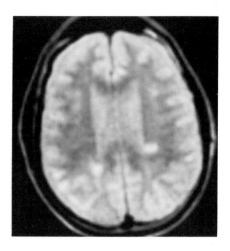

FIG. 36P. SE 2,000/60.

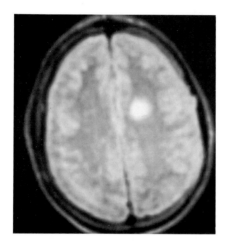

FIG. 36Q. SE 2,000/60.

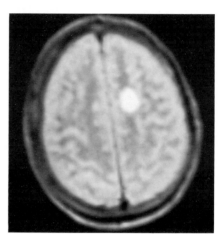

FIG. 36R. SE 2,000/60.

Clinical History

A 50-year-old man initially presented with a three-week history of incoordination of the right leg. Six months later, he developed tingling in the fingertips and the left hand and numbness in the face. Twelve months later, he developed left arm and leg weakness that progressed over 24 hours.

Findings

Three sets of scans are presented, each being obtained after the presentations outlined in the history.

The initial study (36A–36F) is comprised of axial 5 mm T2-W (SE 3,000/80) images and shows a well-circumscribed, rounded lesion of increased signal intensity measuring 2 cm in diameter, commencing inferiorly in the region of the retrolenticular portion of the left internal capsule, extending superiorly within the deep white matter immediately adjacent to the left lateral ventricle (36D, 36E). There is no evidence of mass effect. There is a second 5 mm lesion within the deep white matter of the cingulate gyrus, immediately superior to the body of the lateral ventricle (36F, arrowhead).

The second study is taken six months later and 5 mm axial T2-W (SE 3,000/80) images are presented (36G–36M). Since the previous study, the left periventricular lesion has significantly decreased in size and now measures only 1.2 cm in diameter (36K, 36L). The previously demonstrated 5 mm lesion adjacent to the roof of the right lateral ventricle is unchanged (36M). Since the previous study, a 1.3 cm lesion has developed in the posterior aspect of the right cerebral peduncle and adjacent midbrain (36H, 36I compared to the previous study, 36A, 36B) and several punctate foci, two within the inferior-posterior limb of the left internal capsule, and one within the deep white matter of the right frontal lobe (36J compared to previous study, 36C) have developed.

The third study was performed 12 months later and is degraded by motion artifact. Axial 5 mm T2-W (SE 3,000/80) images of the posterior fossa and axial 1 cm T2-W (SE 2,000/60) images of the whole brain are presented (36N–36R). There is a new 3 cm lesion in the centrum semiovale of the left frontal lobe adjacent to the anterior horn of the lateral ventricle (36Q, 36R compared to previous studies, 36F, 36M). A second new lesion has developed adjacent to the posterior horn of the right lateral ventricle (36P compared to previous studies, 36D, 36L). The other supratentorial lesions are unchanged. Although the right-sided midbrain lesion has resolved (36O), two new lesions have developed in the anterior pons (36N) compared to previous image (36G).

Diagnosis

Multiple sclerosis (MS) with lesions of fluctuating size over a period of 18 months with the development of new lesions and apparent resolution of others.

Discussion

The individual demyelinating plaques of MS are usually less than 1 cm in size, most often between 1 and 5 mm. At times, larger lesions may be seen due to confluent plaque formation, or, in acute active demyelinating lesions, the apparent size is increased by surrounding edema. In this case, the original presentation of incoordination in the right leg related to the large 2 cm lesion situated in the left periventricular region. This lesion decreased substantially in size over the next six months, most likely due to resolution of the edema. The leg incoordination also improved during this period. The apparent resolution of the right midbrain lesion is also likely to be due to resolution of edema related to an acute lesion seen on the second study.

Acute plaques appear much larger than subacute or chronic lesions of MS, and the same lesion may appear quite different as the disease progresses. Apparent complete resolution of plaques may be seen on MR as in this case. The underlying pathology of these lesions remains unclear, although presumably small areas of perivascular demyelination persist.

References

1. Maravilla KR. Multiple sclerosis. In: Stark DD, Bradley WG, eds. *Magnetic resonance imaging.* St. Louis: C.V. Mosby Co., 1988;344–358.
2. Johnson MA, Li DKB, Bryant DJ, Payne JA. Magnetic resonance imaging: serial observations in multiple sclerosis. *AJNR* 1984;5:495–499.

Submitted by: Stephen J. Davis, M.D. and Louis M. Teresi, M.D., Huntington Medical Research Institutes, Pasadena, California; William G. Bradley, M.D., Ph.D., Senior Editor.

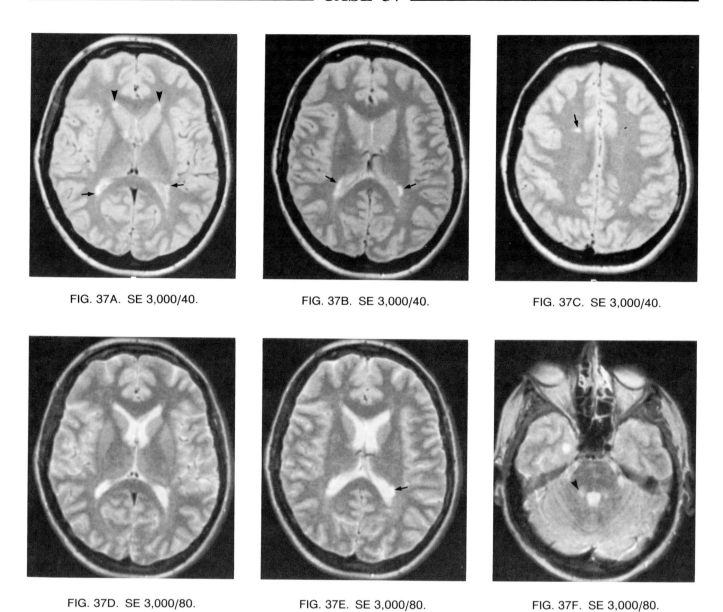

FIG. 37A. SE 3,000/40.　　　　FIG. 37B. SE 3,000/40.　　　　FIG. 37C. SE 3,000/40.

FIG. 37D. SE 3,000/80.　　　　FIG. 37E. SE 3,000/80.　　　　FIG. 37F. SE 3,000/80.

Clinical History

A 38-year-old female with six-week history of blurred vision and numbness on the right side of her body. A similar neurological episode occurred five years previously.

Findings

Axial 5 mm T2-W (SE 3,000/40 and 80) images are shown. There are multiple punctate white matter lesions noted in the periventricular regions bilaterally (37A–37C, 37E, black arrows). There is predominance of these lesions in the periatrial regions bilaterally (37A, 37B), involving the immediate subependymal white matter. There are no posterior fossa lesions. There is an apparent lesion in the midbrain (37F, arrowhead); however, this represents slight asymmetry in the wings of the ambient cisterns that is a normal variant. Metallic artifact from eye makeup is noted adjacent to the globes (37F), and there is mild diffuse mucoperiosteal thickening in the paranasal sinuses.

Diagnosis

Early multiple sclerosis.

Discussion

The distribution of lesions here is typical of early MS. Multiple sclerotic lesions characteristically occur adjacent to the atria of the lateral ventricles and in the immediate subependymal white matter. This is in contrast to white matter infarcts that more often occur more peripherally in the periventricular tissues rather than the subependymal tissues, and more often have a occipito-frontal distribution. Deep white matter infarcts are uncommon before the age of 50 without a specific etiology such as a vasculitis or migraine. (In vasculitis, the lesions are often subcortical or cortical.) Shearing white matter injury may also cause deep white matter lesions, and they may also be seen in patients with AIDS where, if focal, they are likely to represent foci of infection. Lesions occurring in the posterior fossa in a younger patient are strong supportive evidence for MS. There is a predilection for the periphery of the brainstem compared to the more central location of most infarcts, and the middle cerebellar peduncle is also a site of predilection of multiple sclerotic plaques. Up to 10% of plaques may occur in the gray matter. Multiple sclerotic plaques are characteristically discrete and also show a typical oval shape, oriented perpendicular to the ependymal surface of the lateral ventricle along the veins (37C, arrow). This case demonstrates the need to assess subependymal plaques, using the first echo of the T2-weighted sequence (37A, 37B), because, in the second echo, the high intensity of the CSF tends to mask subtle periventricular abnormalities (37D, 37E). Focal areas of increased signal intensity observed at the anterolateral angles of the lateral ventricle in normal people, termed *ependymitis granularis* (37A, arrowheads), are normal variants. Other features that may be mistaken for focal lesions include the bodies of the caudate nuclei as they pass along the lateral ventricle roofs. Other potential pseudolesions include partial voluming of tips of the adjacent deep infoldings of the cerebral gyri, commonly seen at the posterosuperior aspect of the insular cortex. These follow the signal intensity of gray matter, and can be shown to represent cortex by a careful analysis of the adjacent slices. Heterotopic gray matter could also be potentially confusing. Dilated perivascular spaces produce foci of increased signal intensity on heavily T2-weighted sequences but are isointense with white matter on moderately T1-weighted images, the signal intensity paralleling that of CSF. These are most often seen at the vertex superiorly and adjacent to the anterior commissure inferiorly. Other causes of periventricular lesions include infection, inflammatory diseases such as sarcoid, metastatic disease, and radiation damage.

References

1. Maravilla KR. Multiple sclerosis. In: Stark DD, Bradley WG, eds. *Magnetic resonance imaging.* St. Louis: C.V. Mosby Co., 1988;344–358.
2. Horowitz AL, Kaplan RD, Grewe G, et al. The ovoid lesion: a new MR observation in patients with multiple sclerosis. *AJNR* 1989;10:303–305.
3. Sze G, De Armond SJ, Brant-Zawadzki M, et al. Foci of MRI signal (pseudolesions) anterior to the frontal horns: histological correlations of a normal finding. *AJNR* 1986;7:381–387.

Submitted by: Stephen J. Davis, M.D. and Louis M. Teresi, M.D., Huntington Medical Research Institutes, Pasadena, California; William G. Bradley, Jr., M.D., Ph.D., Senior Editor.

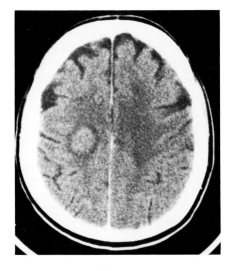

FIG. 38A. CT with contrast.

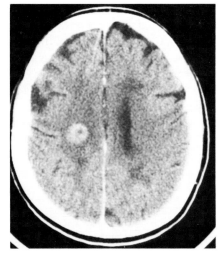

FIG. 38B. CT with contrast.

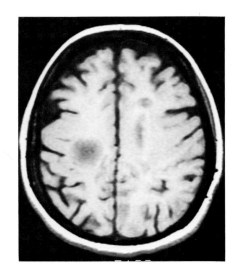

FIG. 38C. SE 800/15.

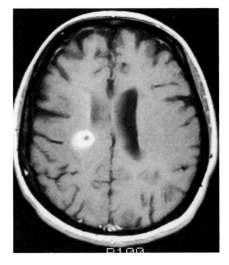

FIG. 38D. SE 800/15 with Gd-DTPA.

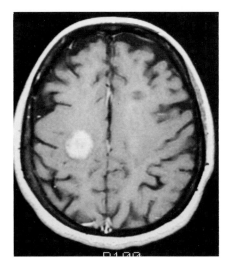

FIG. 38E. SE 800/15 with Gd-DTPA.

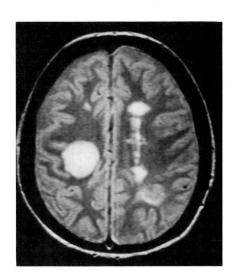

FIG. 38F. SE 2,800/30.

Clinical History

A 34-year-old female was seen in the emergency room presenting with new left leg weakness, prompting the CT study.

Findings

CT scan with contrast (38A, 38B) shows a well-circumscribed lesion immediately adjacent to the right ventricular ependyma, which shows a rather homogeneous enhancement. Note the limited mass effect from surrounding edema on the CT study.

Pre-contrast and post-contrast T1-weighted images (38C–38D) simulate the CT study, low signal intensity shown prior to contrast, high signal intensity after contrast.

The T2-weighted axial sequence (38F) shows the large lesion of the right sub-ependymal white matter, but in addition shows multiple other foci of white matter abnormality in the contralateral hemisphere as well as more anteriorly along the ependyma. The other lesions have a rather ellipsoid, horizontal appearance in reference to the ventricular roof. Retrospectively, subtle white matter abnormality can be seen in the left hemispheric white matter on the CT study as well.

Diagnosis

Multiple sclerosis (MS).

Discussion

Multiple sclerosis can occasionally present clinically and with CT scanning as a tumor. In this case, the CT scan was interpreted as being consistent with tumor—the subtle white matter abnormality of the left hemisphere was not appreciated. The T1-weighted contrast-enhanced MR shows a similar appearance but does define white matter hypointensity to better advantage. The T2-weighted image is rather classic for MS, showing multiple white matter lesions that have a perpendicular orientation to the ventricles. This is in keeping with the pathophysiology of MS plaques, which have an orientation along the transmedullary veins that drain into the subependymal veins of the ventricle. The lesions correspond to inflammatory foci secondary to the demyelinating plaque. When in the active phase of blood-brain barrier breakdown, lesion contrast enhancement will occur. In short, white matter lesions, with trasverse orientation in a subependymal location and lack of significant mass effect or surrounding vasogenic edema, are hallmarks of the MS lesion on MRI. The better sensitivity of the MR technique when compared to the x-ray technique accounts for the improved ability to make the diagnosis.

References

1. Stewart J et al. Magnetic resonance imaging and clinical relationships in multiple sclerosis. *Mayo Clinic Proceedings* 1987;62:174–184.
2. Scotti G et al. Magnetic resonance imaging in multiple sclerosis. *Neuroradiology* 1986;28:319–323.
3. Kappos S et al. Magnetic resonance imaging in the evaluation of treatment in multiple sclerosis. *Neuroradiology* 1988;30:299–302.
4. Brooks D et al. The role of delayed computed tomographic scanning using high doses of contrast material in detecting cerebral demyelination in patient with multiple sclerosis in relapse and remission. *Br J Radiol* 1987;60:295–297.

Submitted by: Michael Brant-Zawadzki, M.D., Senior Editor.

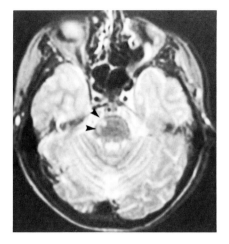

FIG. 39A. SE 2,800/90.

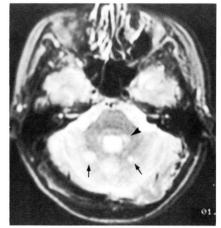

FIG. 39B. SE 2,800/90.

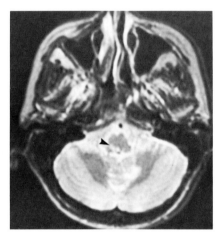

FIG. 39C. SE 2,800/90.

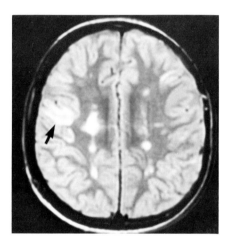

FIG. 39D. SE 2,800/40.

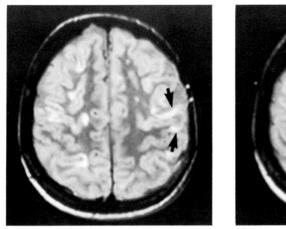

FIG. 39E. SE 2,800/40.

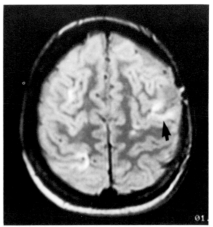

FIG. 39F. SE 2,800/40.

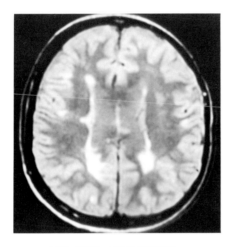

FIG. 39G. SE 2,800/40.

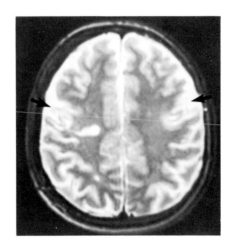

FIG. 39H. SE 2,800/90.

Clinical History

A 49-year-old woman presents with diplopia and numbness in the left arm and leg.

Findings

Axial 5mm T2-W (SE 2,800/40 and 90) and sagittal 5 mm T1-W (SE 600/25) images are presented.

There are multiple periventricular white matter lesions in the centrum semiovale and deep white matter bilaterally (39D). Many of the lesions are situated immediately subependymally and most measure between 5 and 10 mm in diameter. There are occasional larger lesions, e.g., one in the deep white matter of the postero-frontal lobe, and others bilaterally in the periatrial regions (39G). In addition to the deep white matter lesions, there are two cortically-based focal lesions involving the gray matter and subjacent white matter, the largest being in the posterior right frontal lobe (39D, black arrow); a second, smaller lesion is in the left posterior frontal lobe (39E, 39F, black arrows). In addition to focal cortical atrophy related to these two lesions (39H, black arrows), there is more generalized cortical atrophy throughout both cerebral hemispheres.

There are several punctate foci of increased signal intensity in the brainstem. One 3 × 8 mm lesion is present posterolaterally in the right medulla (39C, arrowhead), and two small 3 mm punctate lesions are present peripherally in the right side of the superior pons (39A, arrowheads). There are bilateral lesions in the white matter of the middle cerebellar peduncles posteriorly in both cerebellar hemispheres (39B, black arrows). On the sagittal T1-weighted image, many of the focal periventricular lesions show focal decrease in signal intensity indicating T1 lengthening (39I, arrowhead).

Diagnosis

Chronic MS with brainstem, cerebellar, and cerebral lesions, including gray matter lesions; secondary cerebral atrophy.

Discussion

Although MS lesions typically occur in the periventricular white matter, they may also involve the gray matter in 10% of cases and may involve both the cerebral cortex and the basal ganglia. Involvement of both gray and white matter is particularly evident in the spinal cord. Cortical atrophy is common in patients with long-standing MS. In this patient there is more prominent atrophy at the site of the cortical plaques. Corpus callosal atrophy is also common, although it is not evident in this case.

The distribution of the lesions in the brainstem is characteristic of MS, in which the lesions are typically situated peripherally rather than the more central location of a typical infarct. With rare exceptions, brainstem lesions are contiguous with the cisternal or ventricular cerebrospinal fluid spaces. Brainstem infarcts tend to be more ill defined, unlike the more discrete multiple sclerotic plaques.

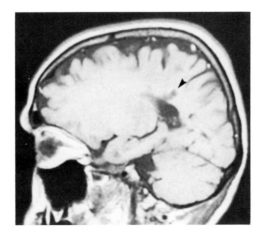

FIG. 39I. SE 600/25.

References

1. Bradley WG. MRI of the brainstem: state of the art. *Radiology.* (In press).
2. Maravilla KR. Multiple sclerosis. In: Stark DD, Bradley WG, eds. In: *Magnetic resonance imaging.* St. Louis: C.V. Mosby Co., 1988;344–388.
3. Brainin M, Reisner T, Neuhold A, et al. Topological characteristics of brainstem lesions in clinically definite and clinically probable cases of multiple sclerosis: an MRI study. *Neuroradiology* 1987;29:530–534.

Submitted by: Stephen J. Davis, M.D. and Louis M. Teresi, M.D., Huntington Medical Research Institutes, Pasadena, California; William G. Bradley, Jr., M.D., Ph.D., Senior Editor.

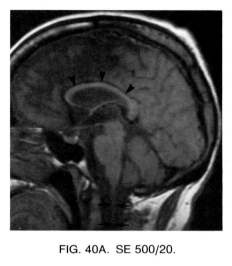

FIG. 40A. SE 500/20.

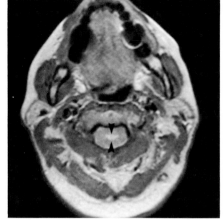

FIG. 40B. SE 2,800/30.

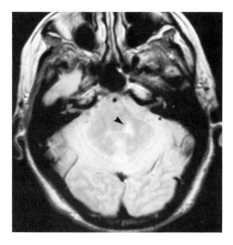

FIG. 40C. SE 2,800/30.

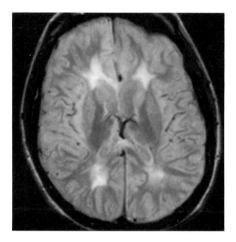

FIG. 40D. SE 2,800/30.

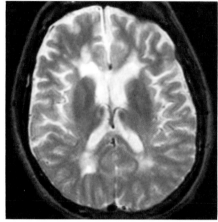

FIG. 40E. SE 2,800/75.

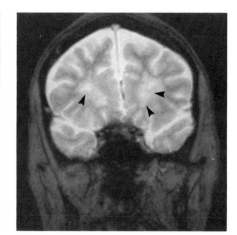

FIG. 40F. GRE 500/15/10°.

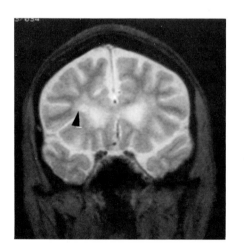

FIG. 40G. GRE 500/15/10°.

Clinical History

A 44-year-old woman with long-standing history of multiple sclerosis since 1976 presents with numbness and weakness in all extremities and progressive visual loss.

Findings

Axial 5 mm T2-W (SE 2,800/30 and 75), sagittal 5 mm T1-W (SE 500/20), and coronal T2*-W GRASS 5 mm (GRE 500/15/10°) images are presented.

Multiple punctate and confluent areas of increased signal intensity are present in the periventricular white matter bilaterally (40D, 40E). There is also an irregular 8-mm lesion involving the left side of the posterior pons adjacent to the 4th ventricular floor (40C, arrowhead). There is marked atrophy of the corticomedullary junction in the visualized upper cervical cord (40A, 40B). There is also atrophy of the corpus callosum (40A, arrowheads) and bilateral cortical atrophy involving predominantly the frontal and temporal lobes (40E).

Diagnosis

Long-standing multiple sclerosis (MS) with upper cervical cord and corpus callosal atrophy.

Discussion

The distributions of the lesions and the corpus callosal atrophy are typical findings in long-standing MS. Cervical cord plaques have been demonstrated in up to 40% of patients with clinical evidence of definite MS, and cervical cord disease is strongly supportive evidence of a diagnosis of MS in otherwise equivocal studies. MS plaques within the cord do not respect boundaries between gray and white matter and do not follow specific white matter tracts. It is very unusual to seen spinal cord plaques in the absence of brain abnormalities.

A gradient echo study is included for comparison. The conspicuousness of the frontal periventricular lesions is less marked than on the conventional spin echo images (40F, 40G, arrowheads).

Reference

1. Maravilla KR. Multiple sclerosis. In: Stark DD, Bradley WG, eds. *Magnetic resonance imaging.* St. Louis: C.V. Mosby Co., 1988;344–358.

Submitted by: Stephen J. Davis, M.D. and Louis M. Teresi, M.D., Huntington Medical Research Institutes, Pasadena, California; William G. Bradley, Jr., M.D., Ph.D., Senior Editor.

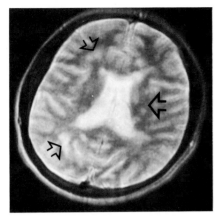

FIG. 41A. SE 3,000/85.

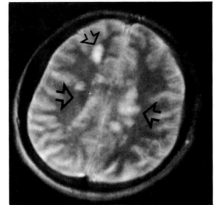

FIG. 41B. SE 3,000/85.

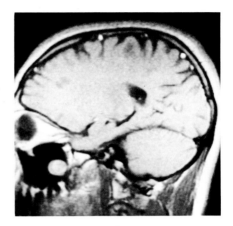

FIG. 41C. SE 480/30.

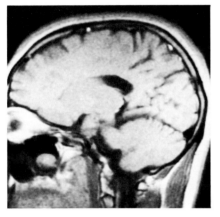

FIG. 41D. SE 480/30.

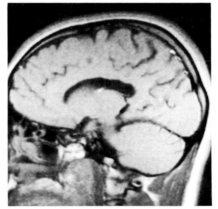

FIG. 41E. SE 480/30.

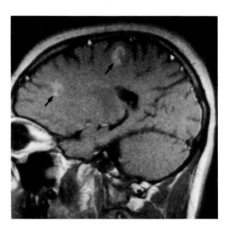

FIG. 41F. SE 480/30 with Gd-DPTA.

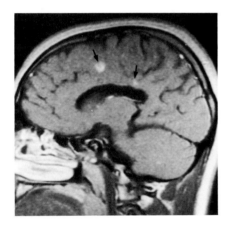

FIG. 41G. SE 480/30 with Gd-DPTA.

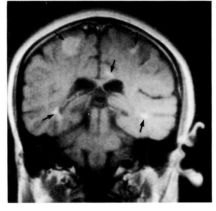

FIG. 41H. SE 433/22 with Gd-DPTA.

Clinical History

A 21-year-old male with exacerbation of multiple sclerosis.

Findings

Axial T2-W (SE 3,000/84) and sagittal T1-W (SE 400/30) images were obtained before administration of intravenous gadolinium-DTPA. T1-weighted sagittal (SE 400/30) and coronal (SE 433/22) images were obtained after gadolinium-DTPA infusion. The axial 3,000/85 images show multiple foci of increased signal intensity in the white matter, with a predominant periventricular distribution (41A, 41B, arrows). Nonenhanced sagittal SE 400/30 images show no abnormalities (41C–41E); however, gadolinium-DTPA-enhanced sagittal SE 400/30 and coronal SE 433/22 images show multiple foci of increased signal intensity (41F–41H, arrows).

Diagnosis

Gadolinium-DTPA-enhancing and nonenhancing multiple sclerosis plaques.

Discussion

Comparing the nonenhanced T2-weighted images and gadolinium-DTPA-enhanced scans, it is apparent that a minority of the numerous lesions seen on T2-weighted images enhance with gadolinium. The possibility of differentiating active demyelinating lesions from inactive lesions in the brain has been investigated by iodinated contrast-enhanced CT and gadolinium-DTPA-enhanced MR. The inflammatory process of an active demyelinating lesion is associated with a transient breakdown of the blood-brain barrier, which is responsible for the contrast enhancement seen on CT and MR. Enhancement has been correlated roughly with clinical activity of the disease. A potential use of gadolinium-enhanced MR in multiple sclerosis is to evaluate the effect of treatment. This is often difficult because of the great variability in the natural course of the disease. The use of serial gadolinium-DTPA-enhanced MR may be of additional value for this purpose when the technique is improved.

References

1. Grossman RI, Gonzalez-Scarano F, Atlas SW, et al. Multiple sclerosis: gadolinium enhancement in MR imaging. *Radiology* 1986;161:721–725.
2. Kuharik MA, Edwards MK, Farlow MR, et al. Gd-enhanced MR imaging of acute and chronic experimental demyelinating lesions. *AJNR* 1988;9:643.
3. Kappos L, Stadt D, Ratzka M, et al. MR imaging in the evaluation of treatment in multiple sclerosis. *Neuroradiology* 1988;30:299–302.

Submitted by: Louis M. Teresi, M.D., Stephen J. Davis, M.D., and Mark Ziemba, M.D., Huntington Medical Research Institutes, Pasadena, California; William G. Bradley, Jr., M.D., Ph.D., Senior Editor.

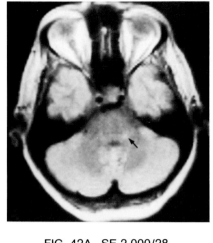

FIG. 42A. SE 2,000/28.

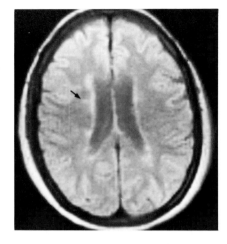

FIG. 42B. SE 2,000/28.

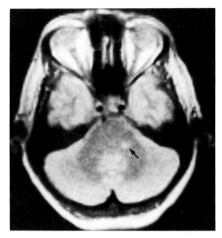

FIG. 42C. SE 2,000/56.

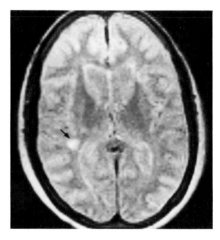

FIG. 42D. SE 2,000/56.

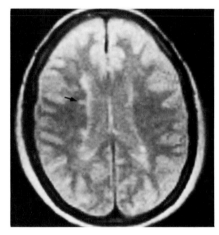

FIG. 42E. SE 2,000/56.

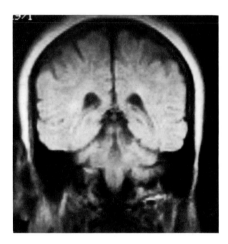

FIG. 42F. SE 1,000/28.

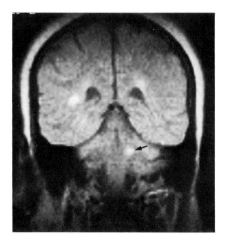

FIG. 42G. SE 1,000/56.

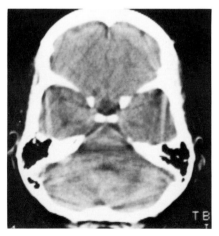

FIG. 42H. CT.

Clinical History

A 44-year-old female with history of multiple sclerosis, now with left facial paralysis. Can this patient wrinkle her forehead?

Findings

Axial T2-W (SE 2,000/28 and 56) and T1-W coronal (SE 1,000/28 and 56) images are provided for review. T2-weighted images show multiple small foci of increased signal intensity in the periventricular white matter, bilaterally, that are most prominent on the second echo images (42A–42E, arrows). Of particular interest is the focus of increased signal intensity in the region of the 7th nerve nucleus on the left (42A, 42C, arrow). Coronal SE 1,000/56 images show this lesion clearly (42G, arrow), whereas SE 1,000/28 images do not (42F). A noncontrast CT examination at this level evidences extensive beam hardening artifact over this area of the brainstem (42H).

Diagnosis

Multiple sclerosis plaque involving left 7th nerve nuclei.

Discussion

The facial nucleus (CN VII) is located just anterior and slightly lateral to the abducens nucleus (CN VI) in the pontine tegmentum. Fibers in the facial nerve then swing medially and posteriorly around the 6th nerve nucleus, creating a bump in the floor of the 4th ventricle known as the *facial colliculus.* The fibers of the facial nerve then traverse the pons, exiting laterally with the 8th nerve fibers en route to the internal auditory canal.

The motor fibers of the facial nerve supply the muscles of facial expression. Lesions lead to facial nerve palsy, which can be either peripheral or central (supranuclear). The most common cause of a peripheral facial paralysis is a benign Bell's palsy that currently is considered to be of post-viral autoimmune etiology. Such lesions may enhance with gadolinium-DTPA. A central facial paralysis is distinguished from peripheral facial paralysis on the basis of the ability to wrinkle the forehead. Such function is lost with a peripheral facial lesion. The visceral motor component of the facial nerve originates in the superior salivary nucleus. These fibers supply the visceral motor function to the lacrimal glands (via the greater superficial petrosal nerve) as well as to the submandibular and sublingual glands (via the nervus intermedius).

This patient's lesion is in the expected location of the facial nerve nucleus, thus producing a central facial nerve paralysis, i.e., she can wrinkle her forehead. Lesions slightly more lateral and anterior would miss the nuclei; they would, however, involve the post-nuclear facial nerve, resulting in a peripheral facial nerve paralysis. In this case the muscles of the forehead would be paralyzed.

References

1. Flannigan BD, Bradley WG, et al. Magnetic resonance imaging of the brainstem: normal structure and basic functional anatomy. *Radiology* 1985;154:375–384.
2. Bradley WG. MRI of the brainstem: state of the art. *Radiology.* (In press).
3. Clark RG. In: Manter and Gatz, eds. *Essentials of neuroanatomy and neurophysiology.* Philadelphia: F.A. Davis Co., 1979.

Submitted by: Louis M. Teresi, M.D., Stephen J. Davis, M.D., and Mark Ziemba, M.D., Huntington Medical Research Institutes, Pasadena, California; William G. Bradley, Jr., M.D., Ph.D., Senior Editor.

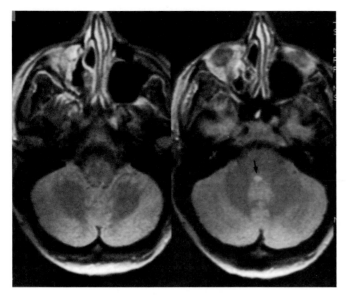 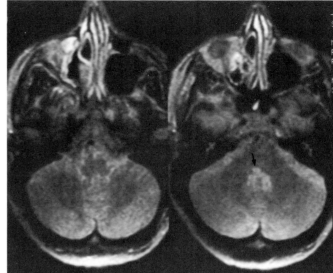

FIG. 43A. SE 3,000/40. FIG. 43B. SE 3,000/80.

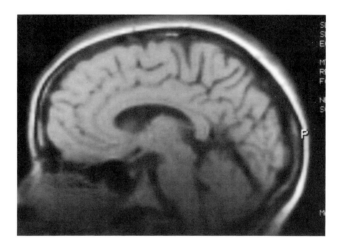

FIG. 43C. SE 500/40.

Clinical History

A 37-year-old female with history of multiple sclerosis and new onset of internuclear ophthalmoplegia.

Findings

Axial T2-W (SE 3,000/40 and 80) and sagittal T1-W (SE 500/40) images are provided for review. Axial T2-weighted images show a small focus of increased signal intensity in the posterior pons, immediately anterior to the 4th ventricle (43A, 43B, arrows). The sagittal T1-weighted image shows no abnormal signal in this region.

Diagnosis

Multiple sclerosis plaque in the region of the medial longitudinal fasciculus.

Discussion

Connecting the 3rd, 4th, and 6th cranial nerve nuclei to each other and to the vestibular nuclei (CN VIII) are the paired medial longitudinal fasciculi (MLF). Lesions of the MLF produce an internuclear ophthalmoplegia (INO). This is a disorder of conjugate gaze resulting from too much tone to the leading eye and not enough tone to the lagging eye as it attempts to cross the midline. When the clinical history of an INO is provided, the radiologist should specifically seek a lesion anterior to the aqueduct or 4th ventricle involving the MLF. The most common cause of INO in a patient under 40 is multiple sclerosis.

References

1. Flannigan BD, Bradley WG, et al. Magnetic resonance imaging of the brainstem: normal structure and basic functional anatomy. *Radiology* 1985;154:375–384.
2. Bradley WG. MRI of the brainstem: state of the art. *Radiology.* (In press).
3. Clark RG. In: Manter and Gatz, eds. *Essentials of neuroanatomy and neurophysiology.* F.A. Davis Co., 1979.

Submitted by: Louis M. Teresi, M.D., Stephen J. Davis, M.D., and Mark Ziemba, M.D., Huntington Medical Research Institutes, Pasadena, California; William G. Bradley, Jr., M.D., Ph.D., Senior Editor.

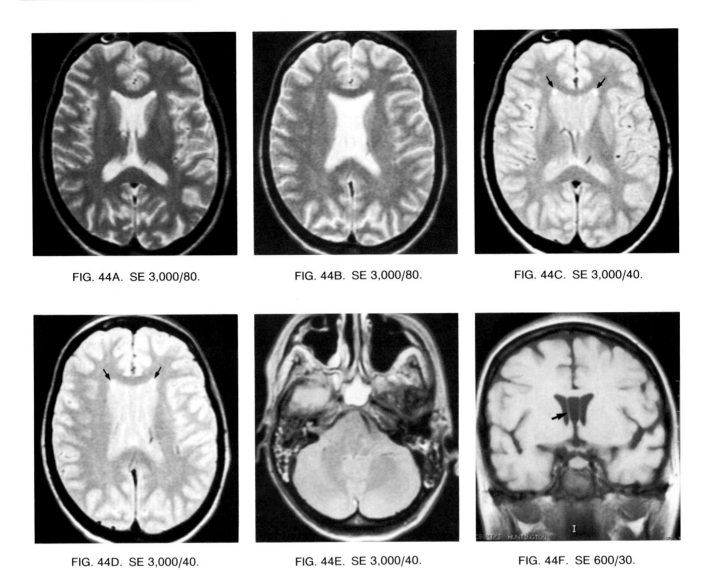

FIG. 44A. SE 3,000/80.　　　　FIG. 44B. SE 3,000/80.　　　　FIG. 44C. SE 3,000/40.

FIG. 44D. SE 3,000/40.　　　　FIG. 44E. SE 3,000/40.　　　　FIG. 44F. SE 600/30.

Clinical History

A 43-year-old female with headache and occasional weakness in the right arm. Requisition states: rule out MS.

Findings

Axial T2-W (SE 3,000/40 and 80) and coronal T1-W (SE 600/30 msec) images are provided for review. The axial SE 3,000/40 images show foci of high signal in the white matter at the tips of the anterior horns of the lateral ventricle (44C, 44D, arrows). These are not seen as well on the heavily T2-W (SE 3,000/80) images as the CSF acquires a higher signal, therefore providing less contrast (44A, 44B).

A cavum septum pellucidum is also noted on the T2-weighted axial images; however, it is best seen on the T1-weighted coronal images (44F, arrow). Fluid in the right sphenoid sinus and mucoperiosteal thickening of the right maxillary, frontal, and scattered ethmoid sinuses is consistent with diffuse inflammatory sinus disease.

Diagnosis

Ependymitis granularis.

Discussion

Punctate areas of high signal intensity on T2-weighted images in the white matter just anterior and lateral to both frontal horns is seen commonly in normal individuals. The region is notable for its loose network of axons with low myelin content. In addition, ependymitis granularis represents patchy loss of the ependyma in the frontal horns with periventricular astrocytic gliosis. CSF tends to converge within this region of brain at the "storm-angles" of the frontal horns. All these factors contribute to increased water content locally, which results in foci of high signal intensity anterior to the frontal horns in normal MR scans. It is important to differentiate this entity from multiple sclerosis, subcortical arteriosclerotic encephalopathy, and changes seen with hydrocephalus.

Reference

1. Sze G, De Armond SJ, Brant-Zawadzki MN, et al. Foci of MRI signal (pseudolesions) anterior to the frontal horns: histologic correlations of a normal finding. *AJNR* 1986;7:381–387.

Submitted by: Louis M. Teresi, M.D., Stephen J. Davis, M.D., and Mark Ziemba, M.D., Huntington Medical Research Institutes, Pasadena, California; William G. Bradley, Jr., M.D., Ph.D., Senior Editor.

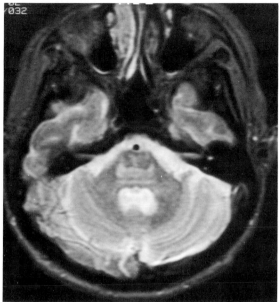 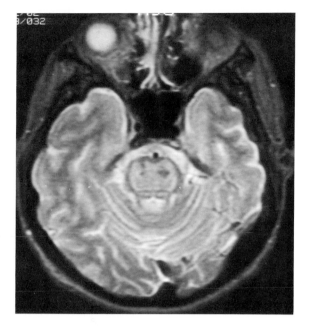

FIG. 45A. SE 2,500/80.   FIG. 45B. SE 2,500/80.

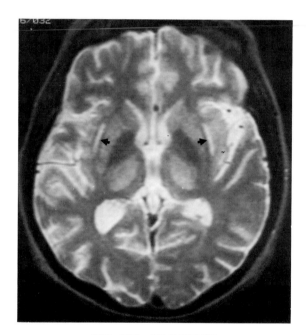

FIG. 45C. SE 2,500/80.

Clinical History

A 45-year-old male alcoholic with markedly altered mental status.

Findings

A symmetric high signal abnormality is present throughout the pons with little expansion of its volume. The abnormality extends up into the thalami, as well as the external capsules on the T2-weighted sequences (45A–45C).

Diagnosis

Central pontine myelinolysis with extra pontine involvement.

Discussion

Since it was first described in 1959, a variety of changes have been demonstrated in central pontine myelolysis. This syndrome generally presents in patients with markedly lowered serum sodium levels, frequently only in the setting of acute alcoholism. However, other causes of lowered sodium can produce this syndrome. It may be the rapid rise of serum sodium from hyponatremic levels that is the culprit rather than the low sodium itself. Lesions may occur not only in the pons but may affect the putamen, external capsule, claustrum, extreme capsule, and the more peripheral supratentorial white matter. Therefore, extrapontine white matter abnormalities should not dissuade one from the diagnosis. Although the disease is often fatal, recovery has been well documented in prior literature.

References

1. Wright DG, Laureno R, Victor M. Pontine and extrapontine myelolysis. *Brain* 1979;102:361–385.
2. Miller GM, Baker HL, Okazaki H, et al. Central pontine myelolysis and its imitators: MR findings. *Radiology* 1988;168:795–802.

Submitted by: Robert Jahnke, M.D., Lovelace Clinic, Alburquerque, New Mexico; Michael Brant-Zawadzki, M.D., Senior Editor.

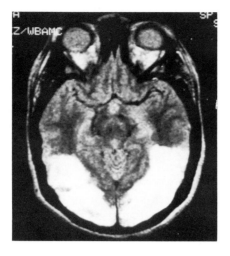 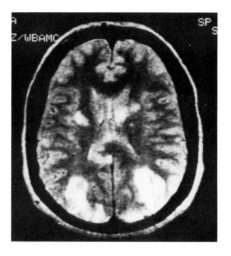

FIG. 46A. September 23, 1986, SE 2,000/63.

FIG. 46B. September 23, 1986, SE 2,000/63.

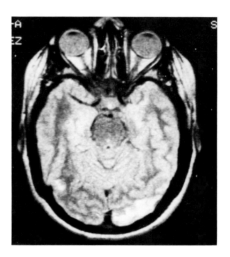

FIG. 46C. October 30, 1986, SE 2,000/60.

Clinical History

A 27-year-old female in the last trimester of pregnancy with acute onset of blindness.

Findings

T2-weighted images at the level of the temporal-occipital lobes (46A) as well as the ventricles (46B) show diffuse signal intensity in the posterior temporal-occipital region bilaterally, extending up to the high posterior cerebral artery distribution, as well as in the basal ganglia. The patient has carried the diagnosis of eclampsia up to this time, with elevation of blood pressure. Following blood pressure management, the visual abnormalities resolved. The scan obtained five weeks later shows only a small area of residual high signal abnormality in the left occipital pole (46C).

Diagnosis

Eclampsia-induced brain edema.

Discussion

The etiology of brain insult with eclampsia remains uncertain, but suggested factors include cerebral vasospasm, hemorrhage, ischemia, edema, and hypertensive encephalopathy. The presentation can be that of convulsions, or focal neurologic deficit of an acute onset. Previous reports have documented by MR the reversibility of the lesions associated with eclampsia. This is one such example.

References

1. Schwaighofer BW, Hesselink JR, Healy ME. MR demonstration of reversible brain abnormalities in eclampsia. *J Comput Assist Tomogr* 1989;13:310–312.
2. Dierckx I, Apple B. MR findings in eclampsia. *AJNR* 1989;10:445.

Submitted by: Keith McMurdo, M.D., Trippler AFB, Honolulu, Hawaii; Michael Brant-Zawadzki, M.D., Senior Editor.

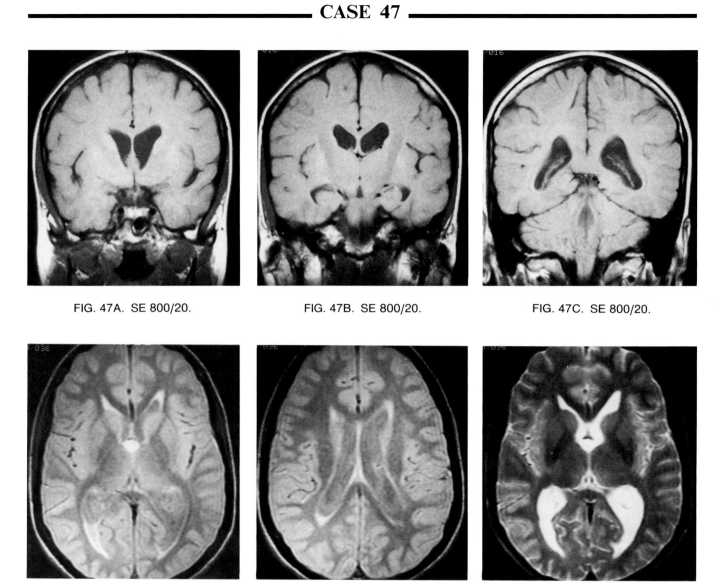

FIG. 47A. SE 800/20.   FIG. 47B. SE 800/20.   FIG. 47C. SE 800/20.

FIG. 47D. SE 2,800/30.   FIG. 47E. SE 2,800/30.   FIG. 47F. SE 2,800/90.

Clinical History

A 30-year-old female with persistent headaches seven weeks following head trauma.

Findings

The coronal T1-weighted images (47A–47C) reveal ventriculomegaly of the lateral ventricles and temporal horns, the tips of which are well shown in 47B. The first echo images from the long TR sequence (47D, 47E) reveal that the ventricles exhibit a high signal border indicating increased water content in the subependymal regions. Also, a small 8 mm round high signal lesion is present at the foramina of Monro (47D). Note the relatively small 3rd ventricle when compared to the size of the lateral ventricles. Also, note that the second echo image at the level of the lesion is much more difficult to interpret, the lesion showing isointensity with CSF on that particular sampling (47F).

Diagnosis

Obstructive hydrocephalus, due to colloid cyst in roof of 3rd ventricle.

Discussion

Normal interstitial fluid that accumulates in the brain through normal hydrostatic mechanisms drains into the ventricular system (the brain contains no lymphatics). When the ventricular system becomes obstructed, this fluid accumulates at the ependymal surface producing the entity known as interstitial edema. This is best discerned on the first echo images of the T2-weighted sequences, where the elevated water content of the subependymal tissue is well shown. In this case, the cause of ventricular obstruction is within the ventricular system —a colloid cyst obstructing the foramina of Monro. The relatively large size of the lateral ventricles is easy to appreciate in this 30-year-old patient; the enlargement of the temporal horns is usually the first manifestation of early ventriculomegaly due to obstruction.

Colloid cysts may show a variety of signal intensities depending on the degree of protein concentration and the degree of polymerization of globular proteins within the solution. Thus, signal intensity on the T1-weighted images may be anything from low to quite high and, conversely, signal intensity on T2-weighted images may be high or quite low—the short T2 occurring with very high protein concentration and polymerization. Differential diagnosis for lesions in this location includes ependymoma and subependymoma. Occasionally, cysticercal cysts can occur here but would be expected to have a much lower signal intensity on the T1-weighted images.

References

1. Scotti G, Scialfa G, Columbo N, et al. MR in the diagnosis of colloid cysts of the third ventricle. *AJNR* 1987;8:370–372.
2. Kjos B, Brant-Zawadzki M, Kucharczyk W, et al. Cystic intracranial lesions: magnetic resonance imaging. *Radiology* 1985;155:363–369.
3. Fullerton GD. Physiologic basis of magnetic relaxation. In: Stark DD, Bradley WG, eds. *Magnetic resonance imaging*. St. Louis: C.V. Mosby Co., 1988;336–355.

Submitted by: Michael Brant-Zawadzki, M.D., Senior Editor.

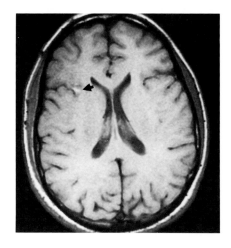
FIG. 48A. SE 800/20.

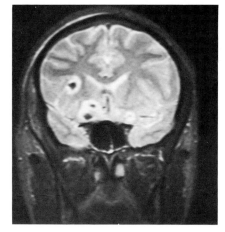
FIG. 48B. SE 2,800/70.

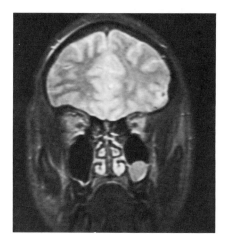
FIG. 48C. SE 2,800/70.

Clinical History

A 26-year-old male with slight memory loss and headache following motor vehicle accident.

Findings

T1-weighted axial image shows a punctate focus of high signal intensity in the subcortical region at the level of the ventricular roofs (48A, arrow). The coronal T2-weighted image (48B, C) shows multiple foci in the subcortical region of the right frontal lobe that contain low signal intensity in the center, high signal intensity in the periphery. Note incidentally the curvilinear high signal over the right calvarium in the scalp.

Diagnosis

Post-traumatic "shear" hemorrhagic brain insults.

Discussion

Here is an example of the utility of magnetic resonance imaging in detecting subtle brain injury. Shear stresses on the brain parenchyma occur with rotational force. At junctions between the gray and white matter, structures of differential density, axial stretching, and separation can occur with disruption of small vessels. Depending on the force, the injury may be severe or relatively mild. In pathologic literature, shear injury is associated with a uniformly grave prognosis, but that represents a highly selected population. MR has shown that small foci of hemorrhage in patients such as this need not be associated with major sequelae. This patient, in fact, left the hospital quite intact three days after this study.

References

1. Hesselink JR, Dowd CF, Healy ME. MR imaging of brain contusions: a comparative study with CT. *AJNR* 1988;9:269–278.
2. Holbourn AH. Mechanisms of head injuries. *Lancet* 1943;2:438–441.

Submitted by: Michael Brant-Zawadzki, M.D., Senior Editor.

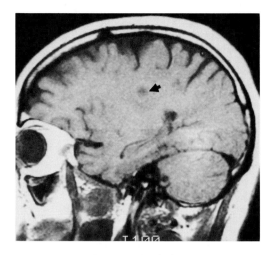

FIG. 49A. SE 600/20.

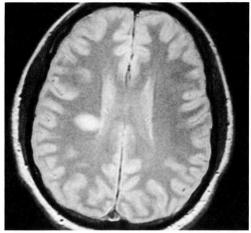

FIG. 49B. SE 2,800/20.

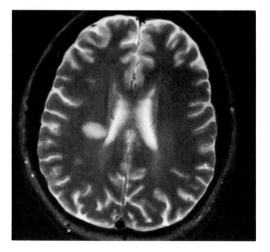

FIG. 49C. SE 2,800/90.

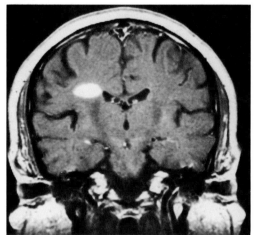

FIG. 49D. SE 800/20 with Gd-DPTA.

Clinical History

A 36-year-old male with a three day history of left hand weakness, facial weakness.

Findings

The T1-weighted sagittal image shows a focal area of decreased low signal intensity in the right centrum semiovale (49A, arrow). The dual echo, T2-weighted axial images at this level reveal an oval-shaped lesion of high signal intensity with the long axis perpendicular to the ependymal surface of the ventricular roof (49B, 49C).

The paramagnetic contrast enhanced image (49D) shows vivid, homogeneous enhancement of the lesion with minimal mass effect on the body of the lateral ventricle. Overall, note the absence of surrounding edema or gross mass effect (given the size of this lesion). No other lesions were seen in the scan.

Diagnosis

Multiple sclerosis.

Discussion

This case points out the difficulty in making the diagnosis of multiple sclerosis on the basis of MRI alone. Currently, that diagnosis must be established by clinical criteria with the MRI helpful in establishing one of those criteria (dissemination of lesions in space). Objective abnormalities of the central nervous system, with repeated episodes each lasting at least 24 hours, and more than one month apart, as well as no other entities that better explain such clinical findings are other criteria that need to be met.

One of the MR clues to the diagnosis here is the oval shape of the lesion and its perpendicular orientation to the subependyma. This correlates with the known pathophysiologic appearance of MS plaques along the subependymal draining veins that also have a perpendicular course.

It should be noted that lesion enhancement in multiple sclerosis has been thought to correlate with disease activity. However, this is not precisely the case. Neurologically active sites of disease may not show any abnormality at all on MR. On the other hand, actively enhancing lesions in the brain may exhibit no neurological manifestations of the disease. Enhancement simply correlates with the degree of vascularity and blood-brain barrier breakdown of a particular lesion. Enhancement suggests recent activity; however, the lack of enhancement does not necessarily indicate lesion quiescence.

The clinical history here helped significantly with diagnosis. Prior neurological episodes had been documented, with resolution. The current problem resolved readily with steroid therapy.

References

1. Stewart JM, Houser OW, Baker HL. Magnetic resonance imaging and clinical relationships in multiple sclerosis. *Mayo Clin Proc* 1987;62:174–184.
2. Kappos L, Stadt D, Ratzk AM, et al. Magnetic resonance imaging in the evaluation of treatment in multiple sclerosis. *Neuroradiology* 1988;30:299–302.
3. Rudick RA, Schiffer RB, Schwetz KM, et al. Multiple sclerosis: problem of incorrect diagnosis. *Arch Neurol* 1986;43:578–583.

Submitted by: Michael Brant-Zawadzki, M.D., Senior Editor.

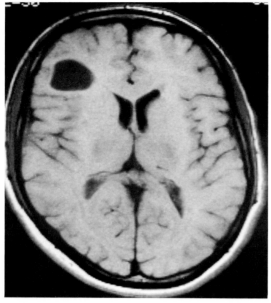

FIG. 50A. SE 500/30.

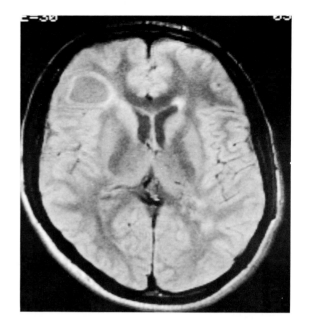

FIG. 50B. SE 2,000/30.

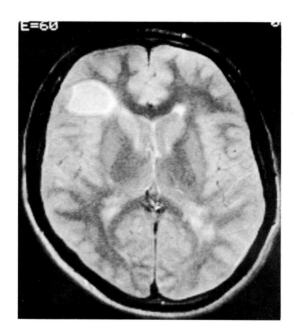

FIG. 50C. SE 2,000/60.

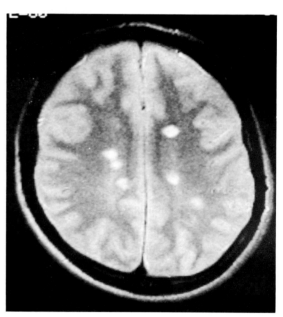

FIG. 50D. SE 2,000/60.

Clinical History

A 23-year-old male with altered sensation, headaches.

Findings

The T1-weighted axial image (50A) shows a cystic lesion in the right frontal lobe. Note minimal, if any, mass effect given the size of the lesion. The first and second echo images of the T2-weighted sequence (50C, 50D) verify the cystic nature of the lesion, the signal intensity of which is just slightly higher than that of ventricular CSF. Note a prominent signal intensity abutting the left frontal horn is seen as well, a less discrete lesion being seen adjacent to the left trigone. A higher section (50D) shows multiple oval lesions oriented perpendicularly to the ventricular ependyma in the white matter. The images obtained three months later with T1 and T2 weighting (50E, 50F, respectively) show decrease in size of the cystic lesion, as well as the appearance of several other white matter lesions in the brain (50F).

Diagnosis

Multiple sclerosis, with cystic component.

Discussion

The cystic lesion in and of itself is a very unusual presentation for a multiple sclerosis plaque. The only clue here is the location (white matter) along with the relative lack of mass effect. Obviously, the other lesions are much more typical for multiple sclerosis and help with the establishment of the diagnosis. The clinical history was quite compatible with it, as is the subsequent CT scan obtained three months later (50E, 50F). Given a large enough lesion and a sufficiently inflammatory response, a cystic lesion of this size can develop and be due to demyelinative disease.

References

1. Wang A, Morris HJ, Hickey WF. Unusual CT patterns of multiple sclerosis. *AJNR* 1983;4:47–50.
2. Paty DW, Oger JJF, Kastrukoff LF, et al. MRI in the diagnosis of MS: a perspective study with comparison of clinical evaluation, evoked potentials, oligoclonal banding, and CT. *Neurology* 1988;38:180–185.

Submitted by: Michael Brant-Zawadzki, M.D., Senior Editor.

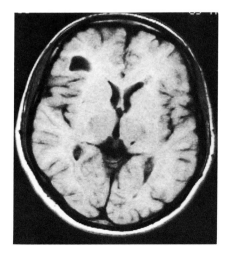

FIG. 50E. 500/30.

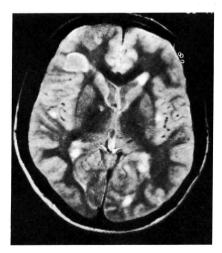

FIG. 50F. SE 2,000/60.

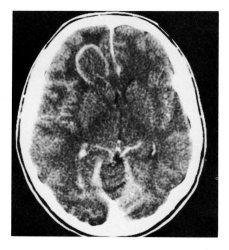

FIG. 51A. CT with contrast.

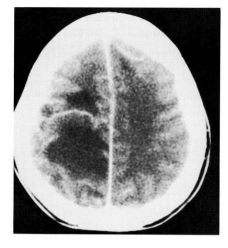

FIG. 51B. CT with contrast.

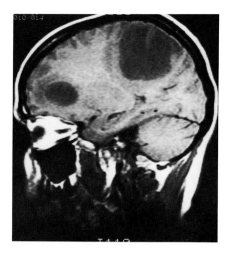

FIG. 51C. SE 600/20.

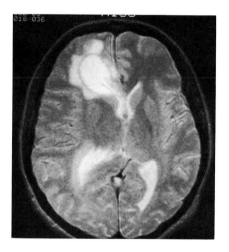

FIG. 51D. SE 2,800/70.

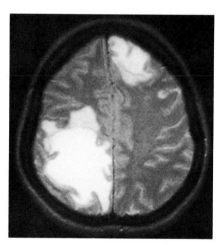

FIG. 51E. SE 2,800/70.

Clinical History

A 40-year-old female with progressive left leg weakness.

Findings

CT scan (51A, 51B) shows very large, enhancing mass lesions in the right frontal, right parietal, and left frontal lobes. T1-weighted (51C) as well as T2-weighted images (51D, 51E) verify the abnormalities with large areas of vasogenic edema surrounding the tumor-like lesions.

The patient was restudied after treatment with steroid therapy seven weeks later. Marked reduction of the lesions is shown both on the T1- (51F) and the T2-weighted axial images, (51G, 51H).

Diagnosis

Multiple sclerosis, tumefactive.

Discussion

Large, contrast enhancing masses with rim enhancement have been described in the acute presentation of multiple sclerosis (MS) affecting the brain. In general, MS presents lesions that have relatively little mass effect despite vivid enhancement. However, in unusual cases such as this one, the lesion may take on a tumefactive appearance with marked mass effect. Fortunately, in this case, the patient had had a prior history of similar attacks; an MR of the spine three years previously revealed a plaque that resolved. Therefore, the diagnosis of MS had already been entertained and, in fact, established with CSF sampling.

References

1. Nelson MJ, Miller SL, McLain W, et al. Multiple sclerosis: large plaque causing mass effect and ring sign. *J Comput Assist Tomogr* 1981;5:892–894.
2. Wong A, Morris JH, Hickey WF. Unusual CT patterns of multiple sclerosis. *AJNR* 1983;4:47–50.
3. Poser CN, Kleefield J, O'Reilly GV. Neuroimaging and the lesions of multiple sclerosis. *AJNR* 1987;8:549–552.

Submitted by: Michael Brant-Zawadzki, M.D., Senior Editor.

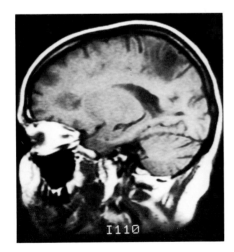

FIG. 51F. SE 600/200.

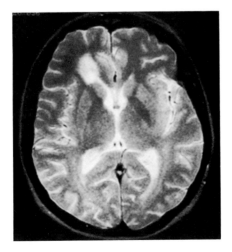

FIG. 51G. SE 2,800/70.

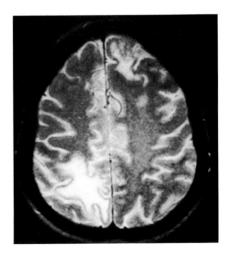

FIG. 51H. SE 2,800/70.

111

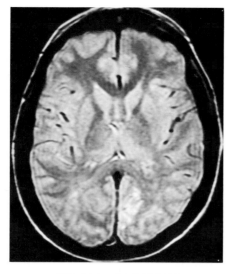

FIG. 52A. SE 2,800/30.

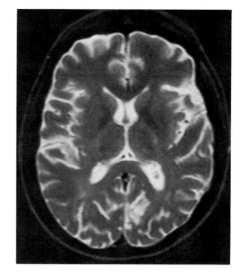

FIG. 52B. SE 2,800/90.

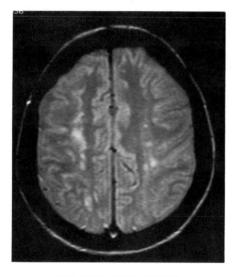

FIG. 52C. SE 2,800/30.

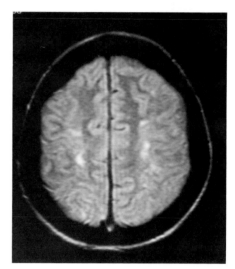

FIG. 52D. SE 2,800/30.

Clinical History

A 29-year-old female with systemic lupus erythematosus (SLE), recent onset of visual hemianopsia. No laboratory evidence of vasculitis.

Findings

Note the gyriform high signal intensity of the calcarine (visual occipital cortex) of the left hemisphere. This is shown both on the first and second echo images (52A, 52B). The latter is more problematic in that the signal intensity of the edematous gray matter matches that of CSF. Also, subcortical patchy lesions are present within the higher cerebral white matter, right greater than left (52C, 52D). These changes in a 29-year-old patient are strongly suggestive of an ischemic etiology with systemic origins, given their multi-focality.

Diagnosis

Lesions of SLE, associated ischemia.

Discussion

Patients with systemic lupus erythematosus may develop ischemic lesions due to a variety of factors. Marantic endocarditis can produce embolic phenomena. Also, these patients have a hypercoagulable state induced by steroid therapy, as well as anticardiolipin antibodies and other factors (1–4). Finally, frank vasculitis can occur due to the inflammatory component of the autoimmune disorder. This is felt to be quite rare, although envoked in past literature as a common etiology. One report suggested that the changes seen with MRI are reversible. This may, in fact, represent very small ischemic foci that proceed on to atrophy rather than true reversal of pathology, however.

The differential diagnosis in a young patient would be based on any cause of vasculitis, including migraine headaches (migraineurs can develop a similar pattern of ischemia and frank infarction).

References

1. Aisen A. MR imaging of SLE involving the brain. *AJNR* 1985;6:197–201.
2. Vermes R. NMR imaging of the brain in SLE. *J Comput Assist Tomogr* 1983;7:461–467.
3. Levine S. Cerebrovascular ischemia associated with lupus anticoagulant. *Stroke* 1987;18(1):257–262.
4. Coull B. Multiple cerebral infarcts associated with anticardiolipin antibodies. *Stroke* 1987;18:1107–1112.

Submitted by: Michael Brant-Zawadzki, M.D., Senior Editor.

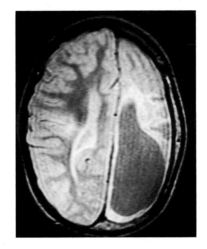 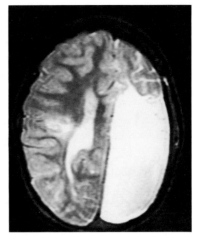

FIG. 53A. SE 2,800/30.   FIG. 53B. SE 2,800/80.

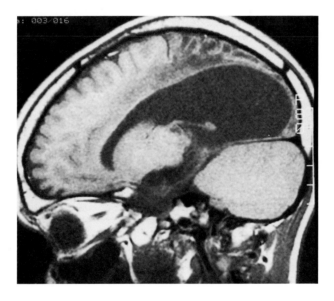

FIG. 53C. SE 600/20.

Clinical History

A young female with right hemiparesis and a history of left hemispheric meningeal encephalitis as an infant.

Findings

The T2-weighted first and second echo images (53A, 53B) reveal a large expansion associated with the body of the left lateral ventricle with thinning of the overlying cortical mantle. The signal intensity within the cavity is that of CSF, as judged by the contralateral ventricle. Incidentally, note also the presence of a deep right hemispheric white matter lesion.

The sagittal image with T1 weighting (53C) documents the contiguity of the large cavitary collection with the lateral ventricle and temporal horn and verifies the rather atrophic overlying brain parenchyma that shows low signal intensity extending from the white matter into the immediate cortical mantle.

Diagnosis

Left porencephalic cyst with encephalomalacia; status post encephalitis.

Discussion

Unlike the case of post-traumatic macrocystic encephalomalacia, where the cysts did not appear to communicate with the ventricle, this is the typical appearance of a true porencephaly —that is, a cavity produced by an expanded ventricle due to overlying brain atrophy. The atrophic picture of the brain is well delineated on these images, with loss of substance and marked elevation of water content within the remnant atrophied brain. This is evidenced by low signal intensity on the T1-weighted sequences and elevation of signal intensity on the T2-weighted sequences.

References

1. Le Count ER, Semerck CB. Porencephaly. *Schweiz Arch Neurol Psychiatr* 1925;14:365–383.
2. Ramsey RG, Huckman MS. Computed tomography porencephaly and other cerebrospinal fluid-containing lesions. *Radiology* 1977;123:73–77.
3. Brant-Zawadzki MN, Bartkowski H, Ortendahl DA, et al. NMR in experimental and clinical cerebral edema. *Noninvas Med Imag* 1984;1:43–47.

Submitted by: Michael Brant-Zawadzki, M.D., Senior Editor.

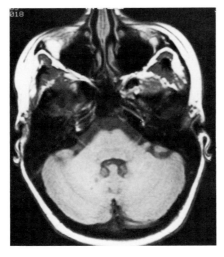

FIG. 54A. SE 700/20.

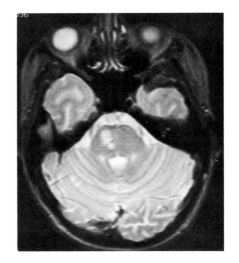

FIG. 54B. SE 2,800/70.

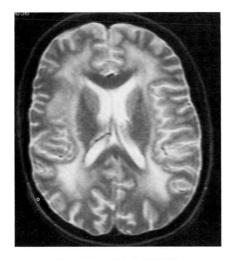

FIG. 54C. SE 2,800/70.

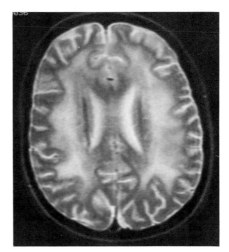

FIG. 54D. SE 2,800/70.

Clinical History

An 18-year-old female, status post prophylactic radiation for acute myelogenous leukemia.

Findings

Axial images at the level of the pons (54A, 54B) show alteration of signal intensity in the paramedian pontine belly only on the T2-weighted study. Higher sections show diffuse elevation of signal intensity throughout the deep hemispheric white matter (54C, 54D). Note the homogeneous appearance of the altered white matter with fading edges and the lack of mass effect.

Diagnosis

Post-radiation therapy, intrathecal methotrexate leukoencephalopathy (diffuse necrotizing leukoencephalopathy).

Discussion

Because the central nervous system appears to serve as a sanctuary for leukemic cells in the face of systemic treatment, institution of specific central nervous system prophylaxis with radiation therapy and intrathecal methotrexate was begun. Occasional neurotoxicity can be observed in these patients. One of the most serious complications is a progressive leukoencephalopathy, the clinical manifestations of which include confusion, somnolence, ataxia, spasticity, seizures, dementia, and even coma and death. The particular use of methotrexate is associated with this leukoencephalopathic syndrome.

However, the heightened sensitivity of MR to minor alterations of white matter has shown that preclinical or subclinical lesions related to either radiation therapy alone or the combination of radiation therapy and methotrexate can occur. Even CT scanning can detect such abnormalities. An early CT study in asymptomatic children treated with radiation in intrathecal therapy showed an incidence of abnormalities in 53% of such symptomatic patients. Therefore, the finding of abnormality in the white matter on MR does not necessarily herald the grave prognosis that the progressive leukoencephalopathic syndrome discussed above can produce. Focal lesions (such as the one shown in the pons here) are somewhat more worrisome, however. These can be related to radiation therapy and may produce focal neurologic signs as well.

References

1. Peylan-Ramun N, Poplack DG, Pizzo PA, et al. Abnormal CT scans of the brain in asymptomatic children with acute lymphocytic leukemia after prophylactic treatment of the central nervous system with radiation and intrathecal chemotherapy. *N Engl J Med* 1978;298:15:815–818.
2. Wendling LR, Bleyer WA, DiChiro G, et al. Transient, severe periventricular hypodensity after leukemic prophylaxis with cranial irradiation and intrathecal methotrexate. *J Comput Assist Tomogr* 1978;2:502–505.
3. Dooms GC, Hecht S, Brant-Zawadzki M, et al. Brain radiation lesions: MR imaging. *Radiology* 1986;158:149–155.
4. Tsuruda JS, Kortman KE, Bradley WG, et al. Radiation effects on cerebral white matter: MR evaluation. *AJNR* 1987;8:431–437.

Submitted by: Walter Kucharczyk, M.D., Toronto General Hospital, Toronto, Canada; Michael Brant-Zawadzki, M.D., Senior Editor.

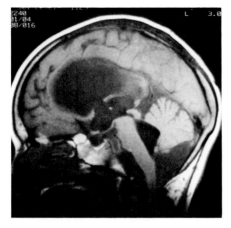

FIG. 55A. SE 600/24.

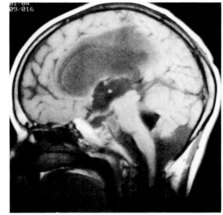

FIG. 55B. SE 600/24.

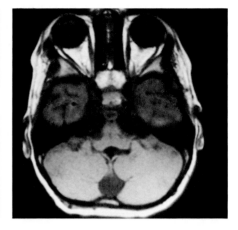

FIG. 55C. SE 600/24.

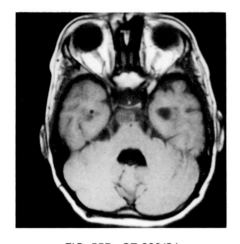

FIG. 55D. SE 600/24.

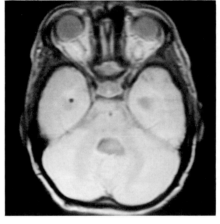

FIG. 55E. SE 2,500/40.

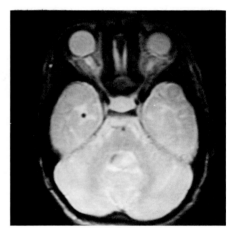

FIG. 55F. SE 2,500/80.

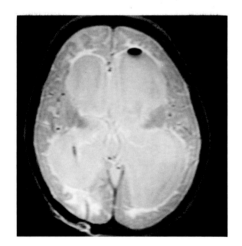

FIG. 55G. 2,500/80.

Clinical History

A young male with leukemia, meningitis, and resulting hydrocephalus.

Findings

The sagittal (55A, 55B) and axial (55C, 55D) T1-weighted images demonstrate a focal mass in the prepontine space, which contains an isointense border and a low intensity center. Note the difficulty in detecting this prepontine mass on the dual echo axial sequences (55E, 55F). Incidentally noted is distention of the ventricular system (55G), with marked dilation of the lateral ventricular body, 3rd and 4th ventricles.

Diagnosis

Candida abscess and meningitis with hydrocephalus.

Discussion

The clinical diagnosis of meningitis in this immuno-compromised host was based on CSF sampling that documented *Candida albicans* as the offending organism. The prepontine mass represents a candida abscess.

Although AIDS has overshadowed other causes of immune compromise, it should be remembered that other diseases and their therapies can produce the immunocompromised state. Patients with leukemia or lymphoma as well as transplant patients on immunosuppressive therapy can develop the same spectrum of disorders that afflict the HIV-infected population.

The phagocytic leukocytes are major contributors to human's resistance against systemic candidiasis. Any factor that modifies leukocyte performance could enhance susceptibility to infection. Not surprisingly, leukemics are particularly prone to this opportunistic organism. Focal masses can occur either in the brain parenchyma or the extra-axial space. Meningitis is another form of intracranial involvement.

References

1. Edwards JE, Lehrer RI, Stiehn ER, et al. Severe candidal infections: clinical perspective, immune defense mechanisms, and current concepts of therapy. *Ann Intern Med* 1978;89:91–106.
2. Black JT. Cerebral candiasis: case report of brain abscess and review of literature. *J Neurol Neurosurg Psychiatry* 1970;33:864–870.
3. Iogren EB, Westmoreland D, Adams CB, et al. Cerebellar mass caused by Candida species. *J Neurosurg* 1984;60:428–430.

Submitted by: Walter Kucharzyk, M.D., Toronto General Hospital, Toronto, Canada; Michael Brant-Zawadzki, M.D., Senior Editor.

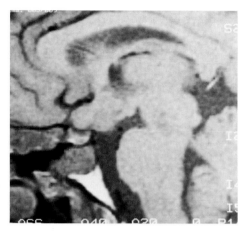

FIG. 56A. SE 550/20.

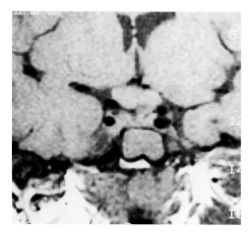

FIG. 56B. SE 600/20.

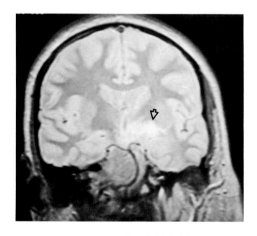

FIG. 56C. SE 2,800/35.

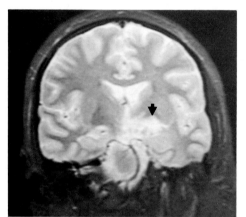

FIG. 56D. SE 2,800/70.

Clinical History

A 29-year-old female with visual difficulty.

Findings

Large lobulated suprasellar mass is seen on the T1-weighted sagittal and coronal sequences obtained without the benefit of intravenous paramagnetic contrast (56A, 56B). Note the obliteration of the suprasellar cistern and loss of distinction between pituitary stalk, chiasm, and suprasellar cistern. Effacement of the floor of the 3rd ventricle is also seen.

The dual echo coronal images (56C, 56D, arrows) show abnormality of signal intensity in the hypothalamic region just to the left of the 3rd ventricle as well. This is a rather poorly circumscribed abnormality distorting the normal morphology here.

Diagnosis

Intracranial sarcoidosis.

Discussion

Note the similarity of this case to the suprasellar component of the same disease process in the preceding case, which was better delineated with the paramagnetic contrast agent. The differential diagnosis would rest between inflammatory meningeal processes such as sarcoid, or granulomatous meningitis, versus hypothalamic glioma, lymphoma, and possibly eosinophilic granuloma.

References

1. Hayes SW, Sherman JL, Stern BJ. MR and CT evaluation of intracranial sarcoidosis. *AJNR* 1987;8:841–847.
2. Delany P. Neurological manifestation in sarcoidosis: review of the literature with a report of 23 cases. *Ann Intern Med* 1977;1987:336–345.
3. Ricker W, Clark M. Sarcoidosis, a clinical pathologic review of 300 cases, including 22 autopsies. *Am J Clin Pathol* 1949;19:725–749.

Submitted by: Walter Kucharczyk, M.D., Toronto General Hospital, Toronto, Canada; Michael Brant-Zawadzki, M.D., Senior Editor.

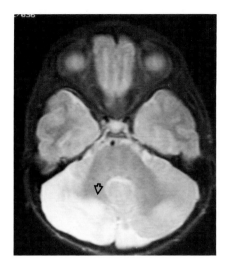

FIG. 57A. SE 2,500/80.

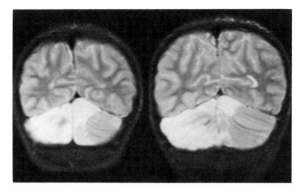

FIG. 57B. SE 2,500/80.

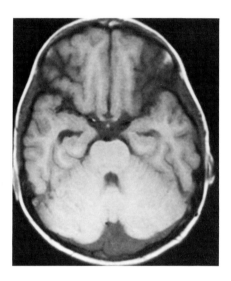

FIG. 57C. SE 600/24.

Clinical History

A young male with relatively rapid onset of ataxia, nausea, and vomiting. Suspected encephalitis or meningitis.

Findings

The axial and coronal T2-weighted images (57A, 57B) reveal a diffuse area of homogeneous elevation of signal intensity throughout the right cerebellar hemisphere, as well as a portion of the paramedian left cerebellar hemisphere. This does not show definite abnormality on the T1-weighted axial study (57C). Note relatively little mass effect is seen, both the gray and the white matter appear involved. (Truncation of the brachium pontis is noted: 57A, arrows).

Diagnosis

Viral cerebellitis.

Discussion

Note the similarity of this case to Case 6. Again, the primary differential diagnosis would rest between this entity and ischemic etiology for this appearance.

References

1. Hosoda K, Tamaki N, Masumura M, et al. Magnetic resonance images of brain stem encephalitis. *J Neurosurg* 1987;66:283–285.
2. Weiner K, Tamaki N, Masumura M, et al. Viral infections of the nervous system. *J Neurosurg* 1984;61:207–224.

Submitted by: Walter Kucharczyk, M.D., Toronto General Hospital, Toronto, Canada; Michael Brant-Zawadzki, M.D., Senior Editor.

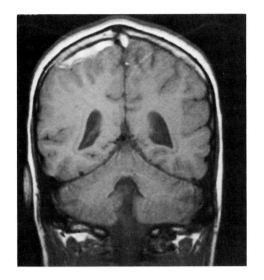

FIG. 58A. SE 600/24.

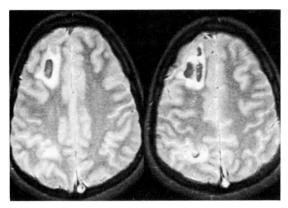

FIG. 58B. SE 2,500/80.

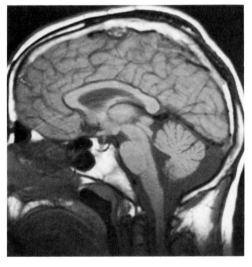

FIG. 58C. SE 600/24.

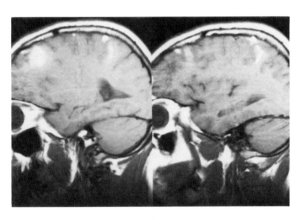

FIG. 58D. SE 600/24.

Clinical History

A young postpartum female with seizure.

Findings

The T1-weighted coronal image demonstrates high signal intensity within the course of the sagittal sinus as well as overlying the right parietal convexity (58A). The T2-weighted axial images document the presence of focal lesions within the right frontal, and parietal subcortical region (58B). The characteristics of the lesions include low signal intensity core and peripheral high signal intensity. The T1-weighted sagittal sequences (58C, 58D) reiterate the high signal contents of the sagittal sinus, as well as high signal components within both the right frontal and parietal lesions. Note also high signal foci of circular nature overlying the convexity.

Diagnosis

Sagittal sinus and cortical venous thromboses with resulting hemorrhagic infarction.

Discussion

This is a fairly typical appearance of sagittal sinus thrombosis in the subacute stage. The methemoglobin components have produced high signal intensity within the sagittal sinus as well as within the occluded cortical veins that would empty into the sinus. Associated hemorrhagic infarction is demonstrated in its early stages on T2-weighted images with the magnetic susceptibility effects of intracellular deoxyhemoglobin (and possibly methemoglobin) producing the low signal intensity. The high signal intensity borders represent elevated brain water. This is a virtually pathognomonic appearance for this entity that can be caused by any hypercoaguable state including that associated with the postpartum state. Other causes of cortical brain thrombosis include meningeal inflammatory and neoplastic conditions, states of dehydration, as well as iatrogenically induced hyperthrombotic problems such as those associated with L-asparaginase treatment of leukemia.

References

1. McMurdo SK, Brant-Zawadzki M, Bradley WG, et al. Dural sinus thrombosis: study using intermediate field strength MR imaging. *Radiology* 1986;161:83–86.
2. Hecht-Leavitt C, Gomori J, Grossman RI, et al. High field MRI of hemorrhagic infarction. *AJNR* 1986;7:581–585.
3. Haley EC, Brashear R, Barth JT, et al. Deep cerebral venous thrombosis: clinical, neuroradiological and neuropsychological correlates. *Arch Neurol* 1989;46:337–340.

Submitted by: Walter Kucharczyk, M.D., Toronto General Hospital, Toronto, Canada; Michael Brant-Zawadzki, M.D., Senior Editor.

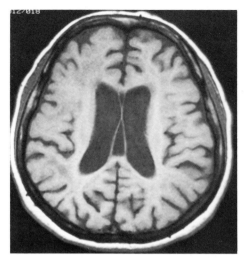

FIG. 59A. SE 700/20.

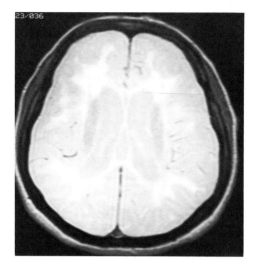

FIG. 59B. SE 2,800/35.

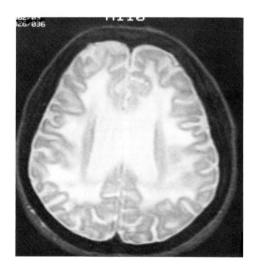

FIG. 59C. 2,800/70.

Clinical History

A 38-year-old female with longstanding dementia.

Findings

The T1-weighted axial image reveals prominent ventricles for a patient of this age, with relatively diminished white matter volume (59A).

The dual echo, T2-weighted images at the same level reveal diffuse increase in signal intensity of the white matter on adjacent sections (59B, 59C). Note retrospectively that the T1-weighted image shows subtle low intensity in the abnormal white matter shown on the T2-weighted sequences.

Diagnosis

Subacute sclerosing panencephalitis (SSPE).

Discussion

The appearance of white matter demyelination and atrophy in this case is nonspecific. A variety of end-stage white matter processes can produce this appearance, including primary dismyelinating syndrome such as adrenal leukodystrophy and global insults to the white matter such as radiation treatment. Other entities that may produce this appearance include the viral-associated diseases such as progressive multi-focal leukoencephalopathy and, as in this case, SSPE.

SSPE is a rare encephalitis believed to be due to the slow virus infection caused by the measles virus. The disease typically affects children, starting with mental or behavioral abnormalities, progressing to include motor signs such as myoclonus and convulsions. Subsequently, the late stages include loss of cerebral cortical functioning. Pathologically, both gray and white matter are involved with gliosis and perivascular infiltration seen in the gray matter, demyelination and gliosis in the white matter.

The diagnosis of SSPE is established by clinical manifestations, presence of abnormal complexes on EEG, and laboratory findings including elevation of CSF gamma globulin, as well as increased titers of measles antibodies in the CSF and serum.

It is unusual to see manifestations of this disease in patients as old as this one. Obviously, this can occur with relatively slow onset and progression of this disease process.

References

1. Takemoto K, Koizumi Y, Kogame S, et al. Magnetic resonance imaging of subacute sclerosing panencephalitis. *Rinsho Hoshasen* 1986;31:999–1004.
2. Tsuchiya K, Yamauchi T, Furui S, et al. MR imaging versus CT in subacute sclerosing panencephalitis. *AJNR* 1988;9:943–946.
3. Jabbour JT, Garcia JH, Lemmi H, et al. Subacute sclerosing panencephalitis: a multi-disciplinary study of eight cases. *JAMA* 1969;207:2248–2254.

Submitted by: Walter Kucharczyk, M.D., Toronto General Hospital, Toronto, Canada; Michael Brant-Zawadzki, M.D., Senior Editor.

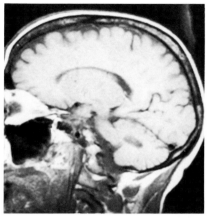 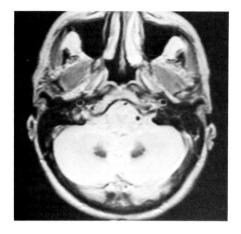

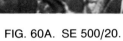

FIG. 60A. SE 500/20.　　　　　　FIG. 60B. SE 2,800/35.

Clinical History

A 54-year-old female with psychotic manic episodes.

Findings

T1-weighted sagittal (60A) and T2-weighted axial (60B) images reveal low signal intensity within the dentate nuclei of the cerebellum. The low signal is particularly striking on the first echo, T2-weighted study (60B).

Diagnosis

Hemachromatosis.

Discussion

Hemachromatosis is a disease caused by abnormal iron deposition in parenchymal cells with eventual tissue damage resulting. Two forms exist. Primary (genetic) hemachromatosis is one of the more common genetic disorders in the general population. Secondary (acquired) hemachromatosis is generally due to chronic disorders of erythropoiesis that are treated with iron and blood transfusions.

The major clinical manifestations include: liver disease that culminates in cirrhosis, diabetes mellitus (secondary to pancreatic iron deposition), skin pigmentation, and hypogonadism. In fact, pituitary failure is not uncommon in hemachromatosis, caused by iron deposition in the anterior pituitary lobe. Elevation of brain iron in those sites that typically store excess iron can also result, as in this case. (No pituitary lesion was found on the MR here, however.)

Overall, increased iron accumulation in the basal ganglia is seen in normal patients of advanced age, as well as in patients in whom the iron transport pathways from the basal ganglia to the periphery of the brain are interrupted. This can occur with severe ischemic anoxic insult or other brain lesions.

Finally, elevated iron content of the basal ganglia can be seen in disorders of neurotransmitter metabolism as well as disorders in which the storage of iron in the brain is increased. Parkinson's disease, Shy-Drager syndrome, and Hallervorden-Spatz syndrome are some of the diseases in which MR has documented increased iron deposition (T2 shortening) in the basal ganglia.

References

1. Fujisawa I, Morikawa AM, Nakano Y, et al. Hemachromatosis of the pituitary gland: MR imaging. *Radiology* 1988;168:213–214.
2. Drayer B, Olanow W, Burger P, et al. Parkinson plus syndrome: diagnosis using high field MR imaging of brain iron. *Radiology* 1986;159:493–498.
3. Aoki S, Okada Y, Nishimura K, et al. Normal deposition of brain iron in childhood and adolescence: MR imaging at 1.5T. *Radiology* 1984;172:381–385.

Submitted by: Michael Brant-Zawadzki, M.D., Senior Editor.

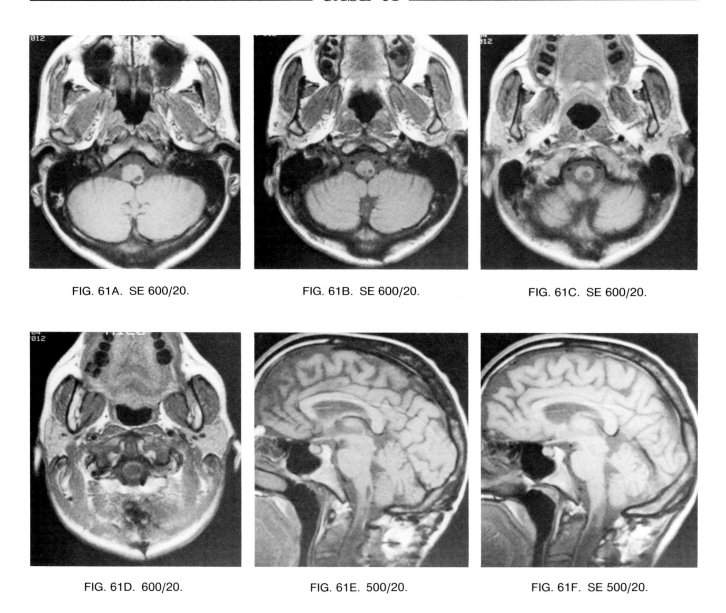

FIG. 61A. SE 600/20. FIG. 61B. SE 600/20. FIG. 61C. SE 600/20.

FIG. 61D. 600/20. FIG. 61E. 500/20. FIG. 61F. SE 500/20.

Clinical History

A 42-year-old paraplegic with increasing upper arm weakness and cranial nerve palsies.

130

Findings

The T1-weighted axial sequences demonstrate an eccentric focus of very low signal intensity in the left dorsal medulla, which continues inferiorly to adjoin a relatively large central cavity in the upper cervical cord at the C1 level (61A–61D). The signal intensity of the fluid within the cavity is quite low, matching that of CSF. There is no enlargement of the medulla, although the cervical cord is slightly enlarged. The sagittal views (61E, 61F) verify the presence of a syrinx cavity within the cervical cord.

Diagnosis

Syringobulbia.

Discussion

Focal cavitary lesions within the brain stem can occur due to a variety of insults. Ischemic insults can produce such cavities, but for the most part, ischemic lesions in the brain stem appear as high signal, patchy foci on T2-weighted images rather than focal cystic "lacunes." Cystic tumors within the brain stem can certainly occur, but they are more often seen in childhood and would produce enlargement of the brain stem. Syringomyelia in the cervical cord can extend by recurrent transient elevations of intraspinal pressure, such as produced by coughing, straining, etc. This extension can occur in the caudad direction, as well as in the cephalad direction to include the brain stem.

In general, with congenital syringomyelia (hydromyelia) the cyst is really the dilated central canal, which is ependymally lined; therefore, the brain stem lesion would also more likely be central. In post-traumatic or other non-congenital causes of syringomyelia, the cavity is within the substance of the cord and can dissect eccentrically as in this case.

References

1. Sherman JL, Barkovich AJ, Citrin CN. The MR appearance of syringomyelia: new observations. *AJNR* 1986;7:985–995.
2. Yeates A, Brant-Zawadzki M, Norman D, et al. Nuclear magnetic resonance imaging of syringomyelia. *AJNR* 1983;4:234–237.

Submitted by: Michael Brant-Zawadzki, M.D., Senior Editor.

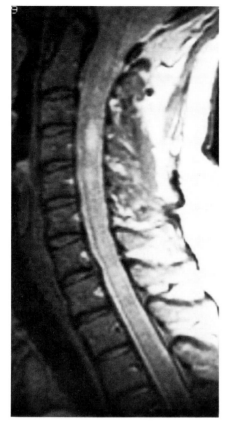

FIG. 62A. SE 2,400/35.

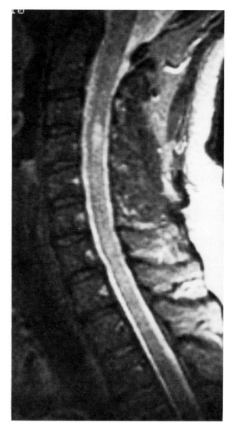

FIG. 62B. SE 2,400/35.

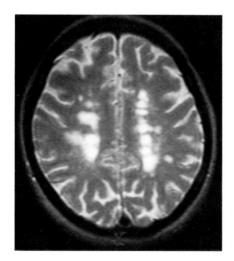

FIG. 62C. SE 2,800/70.

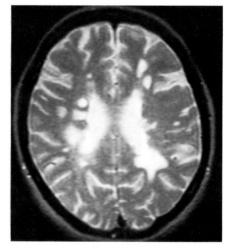

FIG. 62D. SE 2,800/70.

Clinical History

A 49-year-old female with weakness and numbness in the left leg.

Findings

The original study requested was an MR study of the cervical spine. The T2-weighted sagittal images documented several foci of high signal intensity within the substance of the cervical cord (62A, 62B). The brain MR was then performed. Multiple, typical MS plaques are seen oriented perpendicularly along the subependymal region of the ventricular roofs on the T2-weighted image (62C, 62D).

Diagnosis

Multiple sclerosis.

Discussion

This case reiterates the fact that the plaques of multiple sclerosis may be widespread and clinically silent. In this case, it was felt that the spinal lesion was the symptomatic one. Again, when a lesion in the substance of the cord is seen, and the differential rests between neoplastic, inflammatory, ischemic etiologies, one must think of multiple sclerosis as well. In general, in such patients the brain will show the characteristic lesions that allow the diagnosis to be made easily.

Reference

1. Maravilla KR, Weinreb JC, Suss R, et al. Magnetic resonance demonstration of multiple sclerosis plaques in the cervical cord. *AJNR* 1984;5:685–689.

Submitted by: Michael Brant-Zawadzki, M.D., Senior Editor.

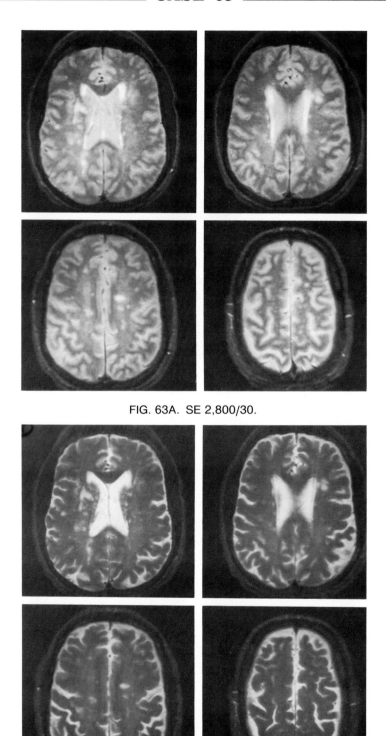

FIG. 63A. SE 2,800/30.

FIG. 63B. SE 2,800/80.

Clinical History

A 61-year-old male with alcoholic liver failure, encephalopathy.

Findings

The series of images from the first (63A) and second echo (63B) T2-weighted series shows multiple foci of high signal intensity scattered throughout the deep hemispheric white matter. These do not have the typical orientation in reference to the ventricles that is seen with multiple sclerosis. The lesions are relatively nonspecific in appearance.

Diagnosis

Alcoholic encephalopathy, white matter lesions.

Discussion

Recent reports point to the increased frequency of white matter lesions in chronic alcoholics. Focal lesions have been found as well as disproportionate atrophy of cerebral white matter in chronic alcoholics. Obviously, the nonspecificity of the lesions makes this a diagnosis of exclusion. In any patient with white matter lesions, particularly one who is below the typical age range seen for microangiopathy of the white matter, the social history of alcohol abuse should be sought.

References

1. Gallucci M, Amicarelli I, Rossi A, et al. MR imaging of white matter lesions in uncomplicated chronic alcoholism. *J Comput Assist Tomogr* 1989;13:395–398.
2. De la Monte SM. Disproportionate atrophy of cerebral white matter in chronic alcoholics. *Arch Neurol* 1988;45:990–992.

Submitted by: Roger Byrd, M.D., Barrows Neurologic Institute, Phoenix, Arizona; Michael Brant-Zawadzki, M.D., Senior Editor.

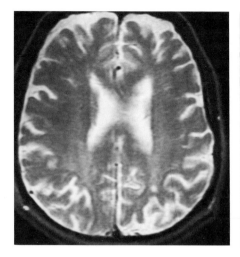

FIG. 64A. October 20, 1988; SE 2,800/80.

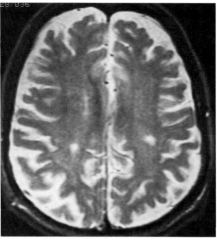

FIG. 64B. October 20, 1988; SE 2,800/80.

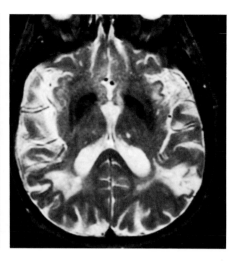

FIG. 64C. January 16, 1990; SE 2,800/90.

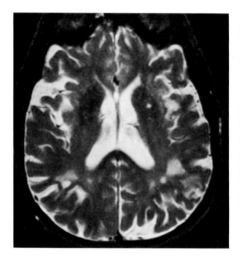

FIG. 64D. January 16, 1990; SE 2,800/90.

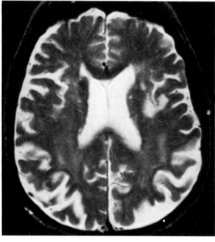

FIG. 64E. January 16, 1990; SE 2,800/90.

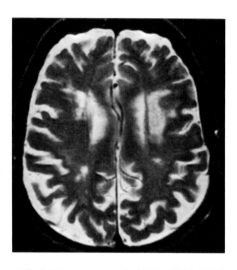

FIG. 64F. January 16, 1990; SE 2,800/90.

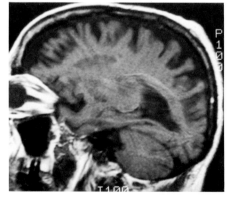

FIG. 64G. January 16, 1990; SE 600/20.

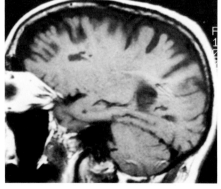

FIG. 64H. January 16, 1990; SE 600/20.

Clinical History

A 75-year-old male with a nine-year history of lymphoma. Patient now presents with progressive mental status deterioration, with focal neurologic findings.

Findings

T2-weighted axial images obtained from a study 14 months previously reveal only two punctate foci of high signal intensity in the deep hemispheric matter of the parietal lobes (64A), with some vague elevation of signal intensity in the diffuse distribution seen on the lower cut (64A). The subsequent study (64C–64G) demonstrates marked progression of white matter abnormalities in both hemispheres' deep white matter, seen best on the T2-weighted axial sequences (64C–64F) but also shown as focal low signal intensity in the T1-weighted sagittal sequences (64G, 64H). In fact, focal cavitary change in the white matter can be seen in the right frontal white matter (64H). There is little mass effect associated with these lesions. If anything, the sulci and ventricles are slightly prominent. No territorial infarcts were identified on the lower sections; the vasculature at the base of the brain showed a normal morphology.

Diagnosis

Progressive multi-focal leukoencephalopathy.

Discussion

Progressive multi-focal leukoencephalopathy (PML) is a disease that develops insiduously in a setting of impaired cell-mediated immunity and evolves relentlessly until the patient dies, usually within four to six months, sometimes longer. Its manifestations are those of multiple progressively enlarging lesions of the white matter. The cause of the disease is a virus, named the *JC virus,* which is nearly ubiquitous among adults all over the world. Under conditions of chronic immunosuppression, this virus can become pathogenic. It is in the class of polyoma viruses. The hallmark of the disease on imaging technique is the demyelinating white lesion with relatively little mass effect and no contrast enhancement. However, the lesion is relatively nonspecific. Therefore, it is a diagnosis of exclusion. It must be considered in patients with the appropriate clinical syndrome—focal or generalized limb weakness, visual field defects, ataxia, and dementia—in the appropriate setting of cell-mediated immunity compromise.

References

1. Carroll DA, Lane B, Norman D, et al. Diagnosis of progressive multi-focal leukoencephalopathy by computed tomography. *Radiology* 1977;122:137–141.
2. Guileux MH, Steiner RE, Young IR. MR imaging in progressive leukoencephalopathy. *AJNR* 1986;7:1033–1035.
3. Richardson EP. Progressive multi-focal leukoencephalopathy. *N Engl J Med* 1961;265:815–823.

Submitted by: Michael Brant-Zawadzki, M.D., Senior Editor.

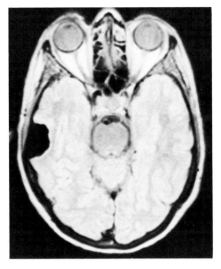

FIG. 65A. SE 2,600/25.

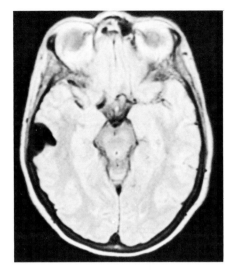

FIG. 65B. SE 2,600/25.

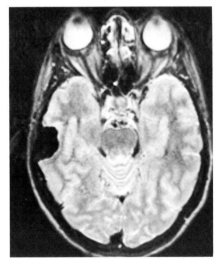

FIG. 65C. SE 2,600/100.

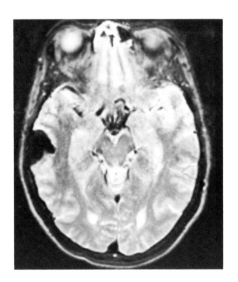

FIG. 65D. SE 2,600/100.

Clinical History

A 60-year-old female with headaches.

Findings

A signal-void lesion is seen arising on the inner table of the right temporal bone on both first echo (65A, 65B) and second echo (65C, 65D) images. No subjacent brain edema is seen. No mass effect is noticeable. No other lesions were present. Similar signal void was seen on the T1-weighted sequence.

Diagnosis

Osteoma, inner table.

Discussion

Osteomas are benign, slowly growing lesions composed of mature dense cortical bone. They can arise from either the outer or inner table. Because of their slow growth, the underlying brain atrophies. On rare occasions, if cortical structures such as the brain stem are involved, symptoms may ensue. The differential diagnosis would include an osteoblastic metastatic lesion, but this would tend to be more centrally located in the calvarium. A monostotic form of fibrous dysplasia can be purely sclerotic, but this is more common at the skull base. Meningiomas generally will have some degree of signal on MR but can be excluded with angiography, as in this case. The history of this patient dating back to 1981 was quite helpful in ensuring that no neoplastic process was responsible for it.

Reference

1. Voorhies RM, Sundiaresin N. Tumors of the skull. In: Wilkins RH, Rengachary SS, eds. *Neurosurgery.* New York, McGraw Hill, 1985;984–1001.

Submitted by: Michael Brant-Zawadzki, M.D., Senior Editor.

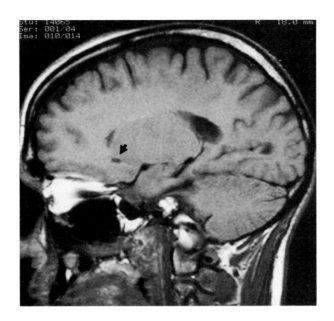

FIG. 66A. SE 600/20.

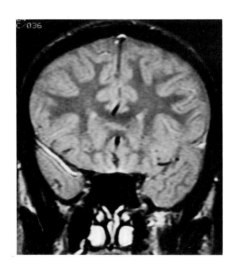

FIG. 66B. SE 2,800/30.

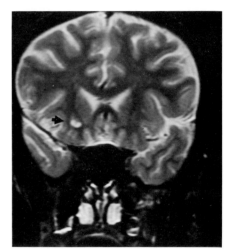

FIG. 66C. SE 2,800/90.

Clinical History

Young male with headaches.

Findings

T1-weighted sagittal sequence (66A) reveals a small, oval lesion with very low signal intensity in the posterior right frontal region (arrow). The dual echo coronal study shows no abnormality on the first echo (66B) image, but the second echo image through this region demonstrates the lesion as a high signal focus (66C, arrow). Note the lack of surrounding edema.

Diagnosis

Benign intraparenchymal brain cyst.

Discussion

Many types of non-neoplastic intracranial cysts have been described. A cyst can form following any brain insult such as ischemia, hemorrhage, trauma, or infection. The affected brain parenchyma is destroyed and becomes passively filled with cerebral spinal fluid. Developmental cysts can occur when a region of the brain does not grow fully, but, even beyond these causes, a variety of other benign cysts can form within the brain parenchyma. In the fetus, transient cyst formation may occur in the developing corpus striatum and between the ependyma and mantle zones of the rhombic region. Subependymal cysts have been described in newborn infants. These cavities can be bordered by a thick glial network. Also, intraparenchymal cysts within an epithelial lining can be found in adult patients. Most of these cysts seem to be lined by ependymal, choroidal, or neuroepithelial cells and probably arise embryologically by budding or cell displacement from the forming ventricle. Such cysts are more common in the region of the temporal horn and the choroidal fissure.

The benign nature of these cysts can be ascertained on the basis of their CSF content, their lack of growth over time, and their lack of enhancement (none was seen in this case).

Similar findings can be seen in older patients who have enlarged Virchow-Robin spaces and invaginations of the arachnoid membrane along the thalmoperforating vessels. Very rarely, a relatively benign neoplasm such as protoplasmic astrocytoma and ganglioglioma may simulate a benign cyst, but the fluid within the cyst generally has a higher signal density than normal CSF, which is best detected on the first echo of the dual echo sequences.

Reference

1. Wilkins RH, Burger PC. Benign intraparenchymal brain cysts without epithelial lining. *J Neurosurg* 1988;68:378–382.

Submitted by: Michael Brant-Zawadzki, M.D., Senior Editor.

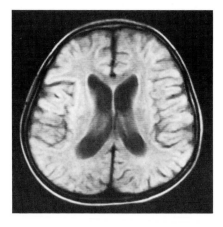

FIG. 67A. SE 2,150/30.

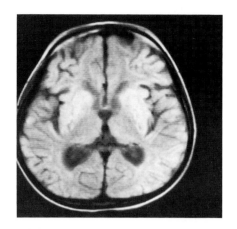

FIG. 67B. SE 2,150/30.

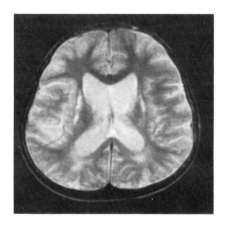

FIG. 67C. SE 2,150/100.

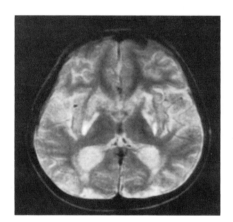

FIG. 67D. SE 2,150/100.

Clinical History

A young male with developmental delay.

Findings

The first (67A, 67B) and second echo (67C, 67D) images at the level of the basal ganglia and lateral ventricles depict enlargement of the lateral ventricles, loss of caudate nuclear volume bilaterally, as well as altered signal intensity within the lenticular nuclei. No other abnormalities were seen.

Diagnosis

Basal ganglial atrophy secondary to diffuse cerebral anoxia.

Discussion

The basal ganglia appear particularly sensitive to global anoxia and hypoperfusion, especially in infants and children. This selective vulnerability of the highly metabolic basal ganglial gray matter has been demonstrated both experimentally and in clinical instances. Other causes of selective basal ganglial injury include carbon monoxide poisoning. Metabolic diseases will affect the basal ganglia in a similar fashion, including the mitochondrial cytopathies.

References

1. McArdle CB, Richardson CJ, Hayden CK, et al. Abnormalities of neonatal brain: MR imaging, Part II. Hypoxic-ischemic brain injury. *Radiology* 1987;163:395–403.
2. Horowitz AL, Kaplan R, Sarpeo G. Carbon monoxide toxicity, MR imaging in the brain. *Radiology* 1987;162:787–788.

Submitted by: Michael Brant-Zawadzki, M.D., Senior Editor.

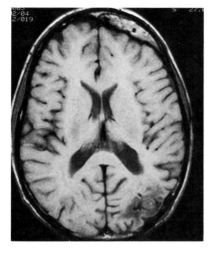

FIG. 68A. SE 800/20.

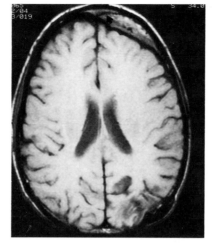

FIG. 68B. SE 800/20.

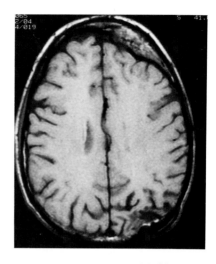

FIG. 68C. SE 800/20.

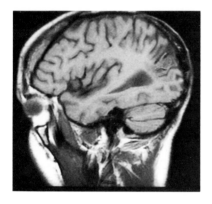

FIG. 68D. SE 600/20.

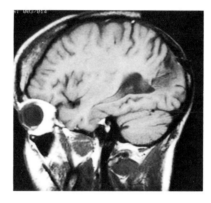

FIG. 68E. SE 600/20.

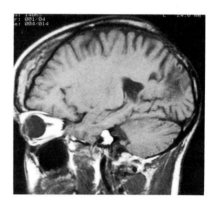

FIG. 68F. SE 600/20.

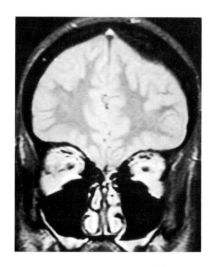

FIG. 68G. SE 2,800/30.

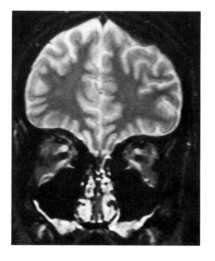

FIG. 68H. SE 2,800/90.

Clinical History

A 22-year-old male, status post left parietal tumor resection, five years previous, now complaining of headaches.

Findings

T1-weighted axial consecutive sections (68A–68C) show an extra-axial lesion in the left frontal region. T1-weighted sagittal sequences (68D–68F) show the lesion again with better delineation of the associated left frontal lobe displacement. Dual echo coronal study (68G, 68H) shows the lesion as well, this time with low signal intensity replacing the high signal seen in the T1-weighted sequences. The CT scan from the period of surgery (five years previous) shows progression of a subdural hematoma to ossification of the dura over a five month period (68I, 68J).

Diagnosis

Ossified epidural hematoma with fatty marrow.

Discussion

This case shows the value of signal intensity changes with manipulation of imaging parameters as a clue to the diagnosis. In this case, the signal intensity of the extra-axial lesion matches that of fat. The inhomogeneity of the structure within is a strong clue to its non-liquid contents. A subdural hematoma could conceivably have this appearance on T1-weighted sequences, but the internal architecture would be more homogeneous. Fibrotic, thickened dura from a prior injury could have this exact appearance, but contrast enhancement would be dramatic (none was seen in this case with injection). Primary diseases of the skull vault such as Paget's disease generally show isointense to low signal intensity on T1-weighted sequences. Hyperostosis frontalis could have this appearance if bilateral and symmetric but should be seen within the diploë. The distinction of this lesion being subdural rather than intradiploeic can be made if one looks at the frontal midline (68A, 68B) where the diploeic fat is seen bordered by the inner table (arrows).

Epidural hematomas, by stripping the dura off of the inner table, may easily ossify over a relatively short interval. If this occurs in a relatively young individual, frank marrow formation can occur as with any periosteal stripping. The history of prior surgery was quite helpful here, as epidural collections can accompany surgery not infrequently. Obviously, having the old CT studies allows easy confirmation of the diagnosis in this particular case. Incidentally, osseous transformation of normal dura can also occur as in the interhemispheric region, where fat will be seen as a result of the fatty marrow appearance.

References

1. Sands SF, Farmer P, Alvarez O, et al. Fat within the falx: MR demonstration of falsing bony metaplasia with marrow formation. *J Comput Assist Tomogr* 1987;11:602–605.
2. Roberts CM, Kressel HY, Fallon MD. Paget's disease: MR imaging findings. *Radiology* 1989;173:341–345.

Submitted by: Michael Brant-Zawadzki, M.D., Senior Editor.

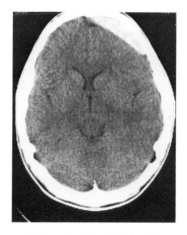

FIG. 68I. July 1984, CT.

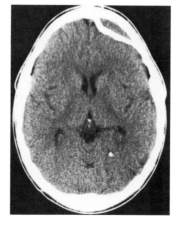

FIG. 68J. December 1984, CT.

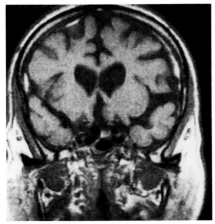
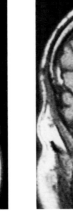
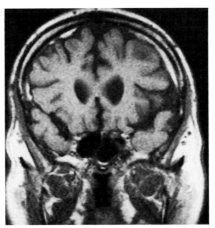
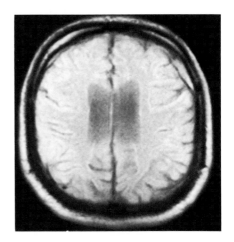

FIG. 69A. SE 600/26.   FIG. 69B. SE 600/26.   FIG. 69C. SE 2,500/30.

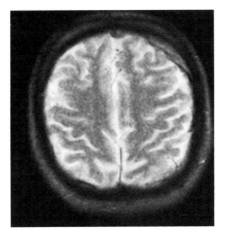
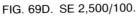
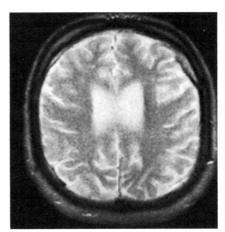

FIG. 69D. SE 2,500/100.   FIG. 69E. SE 2,500/100.

Clinical History

A 67-year-old male with head trauma and headache.

Findings

T1-weighted coronal images (69A, 69B) reveal a high signal crescentic collection over the left frontal convexity, with similar, noncontiguous foci over the right convexity. The first echo (69C) and second echo (69D, 69E) T2-weighted images show the crescentic collections to fade in signal between the first and the second echo. No other abnormalities were seen.

A CT scan obtained ten days previously (69F, 69G) shows a curvilinear calcification of the frontal dura mater. Further history revealed that the patient had suffered a significant head trauma twenty years earlier.

Diagnosis

Dural bony metaplasia, following trauma.

Discussion

The matching of signal intensity of the lesion here with that of subcutaneous fat is quite helpful at arriving at the tissue type represented by the "lesion." The signal intensity of the fat within the ossified dura matches precisely that of the fat within the diploeic fat space. This is unlike the appearance for a subacute subdural hematoma, which would be expected to maintain its high signal intensity on the second echo sequence. Again, the mechanism here for the presence of fat in the dura is much the same as in the prior case of post surgical epidural hematoma and subsequent ossification with marrow conversion. The severe head trauma twenty years previously predisposed to the dural separation from the inner table subsequent ossification and marrow formation.

Reference

1. Sands SF, Farmer P, Alvarez O, et al. Fat within the falx: MR demonstration of falsing bony metaplasia with marrow formation. *J Comput Assist Tomogr* 1987;11:602–605.

Submitted by: Michael Brant-Zawadzki, M.D., Senior Editor.

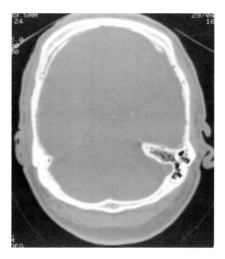

FIG. 69F. CT with contrast.

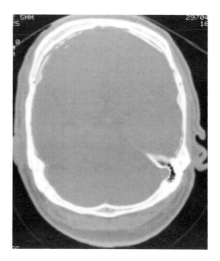

FIG. 69G. CT with contrast.

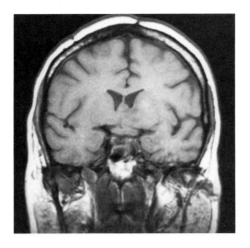

FIG. 70A. SE 800/20.

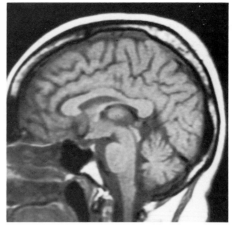

FIG. 70B. SE 600/20.

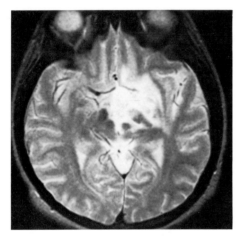

FIG. 70C. SE 2,800/70.

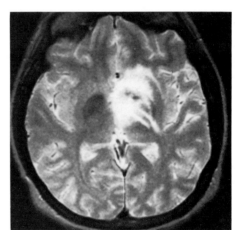

FIG. 70D. SE 2,800/70.

Clinical History

A 34-year-old female with visual disturbance and a history of prior skull lesion.

Findings

The T1-weighted axial and sagittal (70A, 70B) images demonstrate a lesion in the optic chiasm that increases its volume and extends into the floor of the 3rd ventricle as well as left hypothalamus. This is seen to distort the floor of the left frontal horn on the coronal image. The T2-weighted axial images (70C, 70D) verify the lesion's extent from the hypothalamic region into the lower left frontal lobe, hypothalamus, inferior internal capsule, and basal ganglia. Note the poorly marginated edges.

Diagnosis

Histiocytosis X of the hypothalamus.

Discussion

Although the appearance of this lesion is not specific, the history of prior calvarial lesion should raise the suspicion of histiocytosis X. Further clinical workup in this patient revealed diabetes insipidus, as would be expected with any lesion interrupting the hypothalamic-pituitary pathway. Other lesions that could simulate this appearance include sarcoid, basilar chronic meningitis such as TB, and, of course, hypothalamic or optic chiasm glioma. Craniopharyngioma, hamartoma, and teratoma would be expected to have a much more circumscribed appearance with slight differences in localization. Although there appears to be a predilection for the hypothalamus with this disease entity, occasional instances of solitary eosinophilic granulomata elsewhere in the brain have been reported.

References

1. Jenkins JR. Histiocytosis X of the hypothalamus, case report and literature review. *Comput Radiol* 1987;11:181.
2. Penar PL, Kim JH, Chyatt ED. Solitary eosinophilic granuloma of the frontal lobe. *J Neurosurg* 1987;21:566–567.

Submitted by: Michael Brant-Zawadzki, M.D., Senior Editor.

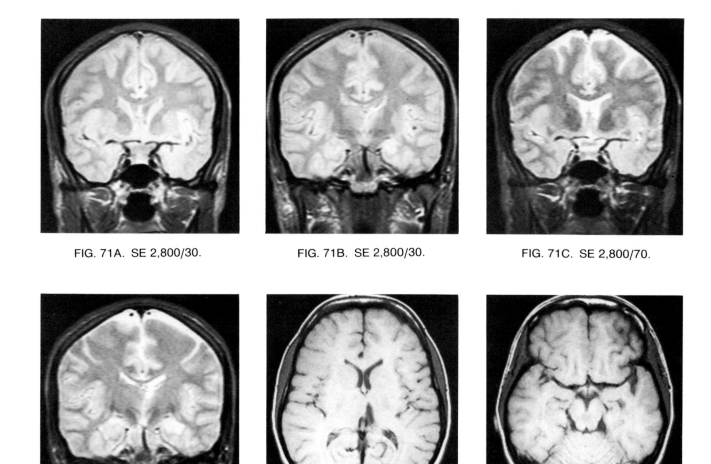

FIG. 71A. SE 2,800/30.   FIG. 71B. SE 2,800/30.   FIG. 71C. SE 2,800/70.

FIG. 71D. SE 2,800/70.   FIG. 71E. SE 800/20.   FIG. 71F. SE 800/20.

Clinical History

A 28-year-old female with long-standing left temporal lobe seizures and increasing difficulty in control.

Findings

The first (71A, 71B) and second (71C, 71D) echo images of the T2-weighted coronal sequence demonstrate a subtle abnormality of the left temporal lobe, specifically in the region of the luncus and hippocampus. Some distortion of the normal gray-white interdigitation and morphology is seen (compared to the right temporal lobe). Accompanying this is a slight elevation of signal intensity shown particularly on the more posterior cuts in the region of the amygdala (71B, 71D). The axial T1-weighted images demonstrate a cleft-like defect adjacent to the posterior third ventricle in the left thalamus, as well as asymmetric enlargement of the left temporal horn compared to the right (71E, 71F).

Diagnosis

Mesial temporal sclerosis.

Discussion

The contribution of MR imaging in patients with temporal lobe epilepsy has surpassed that of CT. Although in many cases the major value is either the detection of mass lesions or their exclusion, in some cases certain specific findings for mesial temporal sclerosis can be seen. This is an example. The enlargement of the temporal horn as well as the cleft-like defect in the posterior thalamus strongly suggest a chronic abnormality from a long-standing insult (possibly an in-utero one). The alteration of gray-white interdigitation suggests the disorganization that is found histologically in lesions of mesial temporal sclerosis. Presumably, the atrophy of the region is reflected in the temporal horn dilatation, whereas the cleft in the thalamic region suggests a vascular insult as the cause of the abnormality (given that the same parental branch middle cerebral artery supplies blood to both regions).

References

1. Brooks BS, King DW, et al. MR imaging in patients with intractable complex partial epileptic seizures. *AJR* 1990;11:93–99.
2. Jabbari B, Gunderson CH, Wippold F, et al. Magnetic resonance imaging in partial complex epilepsy. *Arch Neurol* 1986;43:869–872.

Submitted by: Michael Brant-Zawadzki, M.D., Senior Editor.

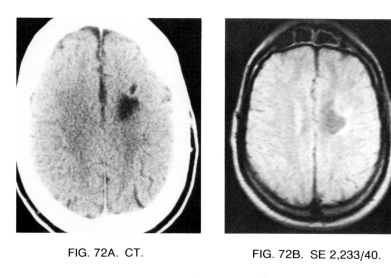

FIG. 72A. CT.   FIG. 72B. SE 2,233/40.

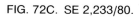
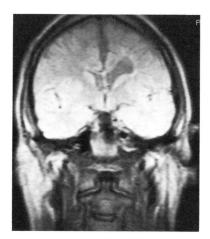

FIG. 72C. SE 2,233/80.   FIG. 72D. SE 2,233/40.

Clinical History

A 39-year-old male, motor vehicle accident, rule out intracranial trauma.

Findings

A CT scan (72A) showed a low attenuating lesion in the region immediately above the left ventricular roof. This was an incidental finding. MRI studies show the same lesion on the dual echo sequences (72B, 72C), the signal intensity matching that of CSF. Punctate foci of elevated signal in the immediately subjacent white matter are also noted. The coronal first echo image of a long TR sequence (72D) shows the lesion to be essentially a diverticular-like outpouching of the left ventricular roof.

Diagnosis

Focal porencephaly.

Discussion

This incidental finding is most likely the result of a long-standing lesion, one that may have been acquired even in utero, producing focal atrophy immediately at the ventricular roof. This may well have been a germinal matrix bleed. Found incidentally in this middle-aged patient, it should not be mistaken for an active lesion. The punctate high signal foci in the subjacent white matter most likely reflect microcystic encephalomalacia.

Reference

1. Kjos BO, Brant-Zawadzki MN, Kucharczyk W, et al. Cystic intracranial lesions: magnetic resonance imaging. *Radiology* 1985;155:363–369.

Submitted by: Michael Brant-Zawadzki, M.D., Senior Editor.

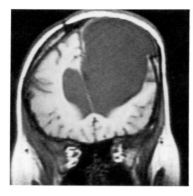

FIG. 73A. SE 800/20.

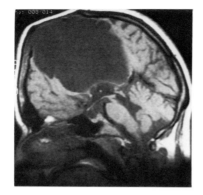

FIG. 73B. SE 600/20.

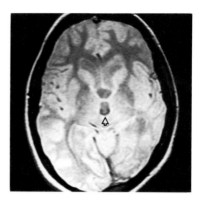

FIG. 73C. SE 2,800/30.

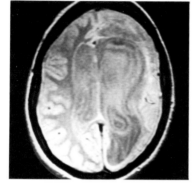

FIG. 73D. SE 2,800/30.

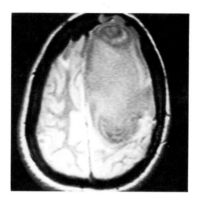

FIG. 73E. SE 2,800/30.

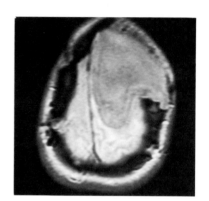

FIG. 73F. SE 2,800/30.

Clinical History

A 24-year-old female with progressive ataxia. Past head injury at age of three months, including left frontal parietal skull fracture, resulting in psychomotor disability thereafter.

Findings

The coronal T1-weighted image reveals a large cyst communicating with the left lateral ventricle (73A). Note the enlarged contralateral ventricle. The sagittal T1-weighted image in the midline verifies the porencephalic nature of the cyst, arising from the left ventricle (73B). Note, incidentally, the enlarged 3rd ventricle, aqueduct, and 4th ventricle. The axial, first echo T2-weighted images (73C–73F) verify these findings, showing the enlarged ventricular system and the porencephalic cyst extending to the calvarium and, in fact, eroding through it. Note the serpentine pulsatile flow phenomenon within the enlarged left ventricular system particularly. Exaggerated signal void can be seen within the posterior 3rd ventricle (73C, arrow).

Diagnosis

Post-traumatic porencephalic cyst, acting like leptomeningeal cyst due to progressive hydrocephalus.

Discussion

The large cystic abnormality fits the criteria of a porencephalic cyst, namely, a cavitary-like expansion of the ventricle into an area of brain substance loss. In this case, the cyst has begun to act as a classic post-traumatic leptomeningeal cyst. Leptomeningeal cysts occur due to inclusion of the arachnoid space within a non-healing skull fracture, the resulting CSF pulsations enlarging the fracture and producing a cystic-like expansion. In this case, the cyst is actually porencephalic in nature, with progressive growth due to an overall communicating hydrocephalus that has developed. The hyperdynamic state of the ventricular system is nicely exhibited by the flow phenomenon described in the findings section.

Reference

1. Bradley WG. Hydrocephalus and atrophy. In: *Magnetic resonance imaging.* Stark DD, Bradley WG, eds. St. Louis: C. V. Mosby, 1988; 451–472.

Submitted by: Michael Brant-Zawadzki, M.D., Senior Editor.

155

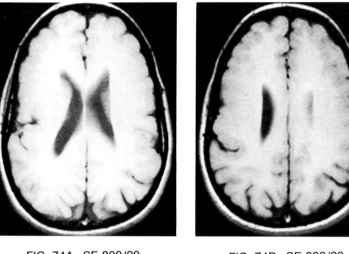

FIG. 74A. SE 800/20.   FIG. 74B. SE 800/20.

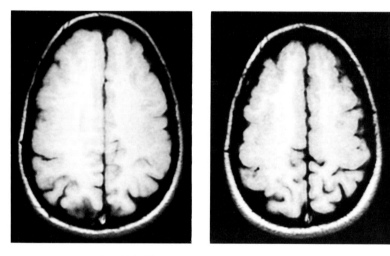

FIG. 74C. SE 800/20.   FIG. 74D. SE 800/20.

Clinical History

A 32-year-old female with history of "cerebral palsy" and recent onset of seizures.

Findings

The T1-weighted axial sequences (74A–74D) demonstrate a striking lack of sulcal development in the frontal lobes, the right more prominently than the left, extending over the cerebral convexities. This lends a relatively smooth appearance to the brain surface.

Diagnosis

Pachygyria.

Discussion

Pachygyria, agyria, and microgyria may show broad, poorly separated gyri, and shallow sulci associated with thickened cortex at gross inspection. Histologically, pachygyria shows disorganized cortex composed of four layers: an outer molecular layer, a disorganized, superficial cellular layer, and cell-sparse and deep cellular layers, both of which are not seen in normal cortex. True agyria shows lack of sulcation. Failure of migration is generally believed to occur between eight and sixteen weeks in utero and the abnormal cortex is presumably incapable of going on to form sulci that normally form after 26 weeks. No definite developmental difference is known to exist between frontal and occipital gyri. However, recent investigations have suggested that patients with nondiffuse pachygyric-like changes confined to the frontal lobes can at times exhibit only minimal retardation and independent function, requiring less care, with survival into adulthood as compared to the severe retardation and poor prognosis in patients with diffuse pachygyria as well as frank lissencephaly. Therefore, on rare occasions, a patient who presents as this one has in early middle age may be found to have a congenital malformation of the migrational disorder category accounting for seizures.

Reference

1. Titelbaum DS, Hayward JC, Zimmerman RA. Pachygyric-like changes: topographic appearance at MR imaging and CT and correlation with neurological status. *Radiology* 1989;173:663–667.

Submitted by: Michael Brant-Zawadzki, M.D., Senior Editor.

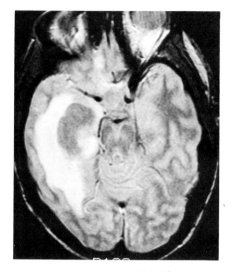

FIG. 75A. SE 2,800/30.

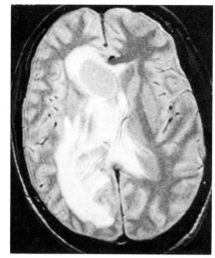

FIG. 75B. SE 2,800/30.

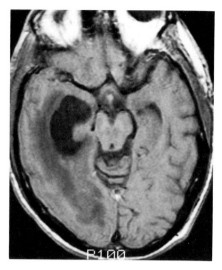

FIG. 75C. SE 800/20 with Gd-DPTA.

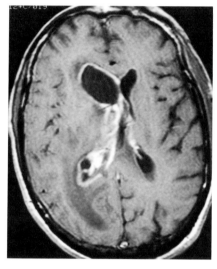

FIG. 75D. SE 800/20 with Gd-DPTA.

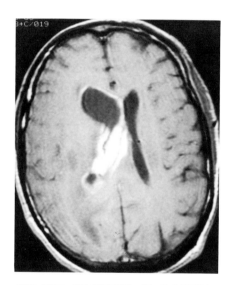

FIG. 75E. SE 800/20 with Gd-DPTA.

Clinical History

A 39-year-old male with AIDS and altered mental status.

Findings

The first echo images from the long TR sequence (75A, 75B) reveal a large amount of edema surrounding the dilated left ventricular system, crossing the splenium of the corpus callosum. The gadolinium-DTPA-enhanced T1-weighted axial images (75C–75E) verify the enlarged right ventricular system and show contrast enhancement bordering the ependyma of the entire lateral ventricle, with a more concentrated area of enhancement seen at the ventricular-callosal interface posteriorly (75E). Note the lack of contralateral ventricular dilatation.

Diagnosis

Trapped ventricle, secondary to lymphoma.

Discussion

Unilateral ventricular enlargement can occur any time that the choroid-producing segment of a ventricle is trapped. Continued CSF production in the absence of communication with the remnant ventricular system produces focal ventriculomegaly as in this case. The interstitial edema that develops surrounding the ventricular system in any case of obstructive hydrocephalus may become quite extensive in cases with a focally obstructed ventricular system where frank disruption of the ependymal lining occurs with egress of intraventricular CSF into the surrounding subependymal region. This is particularly the case when an aggravating lesion such as infection or tumor produces this abnormality. It has been said that vasogenic edema (edema of the white matter) does not generally cross the corpus callosum due to the heavily myelinated, closely apposed white matter tracts there. In this case, however, the lesion itself is in the corpus callosum, thus producing the edema shown in the splenium.

Reference

1. Bradley WG. Hydrocephalus and atrophy. In: *Magnetic resonance imaging.* Stark DD, Bradley WG, eds. St. Louis: C. V. Mosby, 1988; 451–472.

Submitted by: Michael Brant-Zawadzki, M.D., Senior Editor.

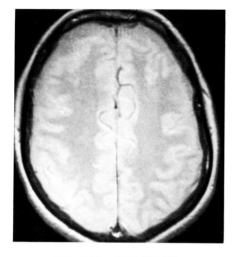

FIG. 76A. SE 2,800/30.

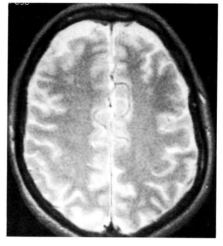

FIG. 76B. SE 2,800/70.

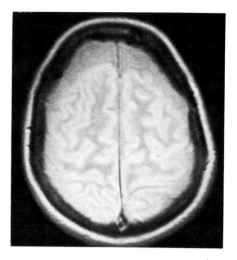

FIG. 76C. SE 2,800/30.

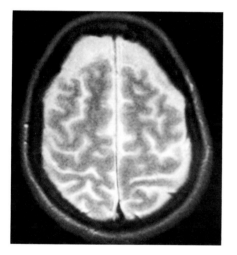

FIG. 76D. SE 2,800/70.

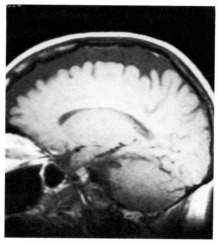

FIG. 76E. SE 600/20.

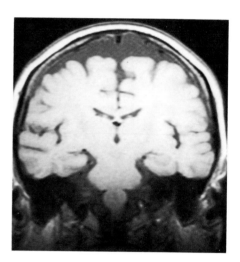

FIG. 76F. SE 600/20.

Clinical History

A 58-year-old female with seizures.

Findings

The dual echo pairs of images (76A–76D) suggest the presence of prefrontal fluid collections with CSF-consistency over the convexity. The T1-weighted sagittal and coronal images (76E, 76F) verify prominent fluid collections overlying both convexities, particularly notable in the midline.

Diagnosis

Subdural chronic hygroma.

Discussion

"Silent" subdural hygromas occur with some frequency following head injury. These subdural hygromas tend to show a crescentic extracerebral collection with some preservation of major sulci and frequently produce interhemispheric fluid as well. The mechanism is thought to be due to a tear in the arachnoid that then functions as a one-way valve allowing cerebrospinal fluid to enter the subdural space and to be trapped with little or no absorption. However, the mechanism of the development of subdural fluid hygromas is not fully understood. In the absence of history of significant trauma, one might wonder if these collections are really representative of brain atrophy. However, in this case, the relatively small size of the ventricular system and the sulci argue strongly against the presence of atrophy, particularly in the localized convexity region where the hygroma appears. Occasionally, even relatively minor head trauma can produce such accumulations.

Reference

1. Masuzawa T, Kumagai M, Sato F, et al. Computed tomographic evolution of post-traumatic subdural hygroma in young adults. *Neuroradiology* 1984;26:245–248.

Submitted by: Michael Brant-Zawadzki, M.D., Senior Editor.

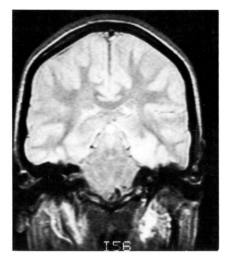

FIG. 77A. 1990, SE 2,800/30.

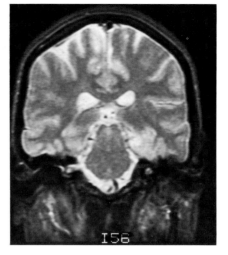

FIG. 77B. 1990, SE 2,800/70.

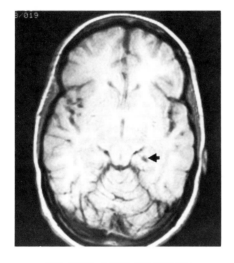

FIG. 77C. 1990, SE 800/20.

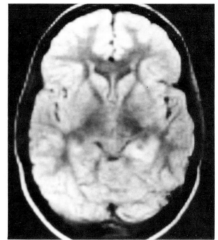

FIG. 77D. 1985, SE 2,000/28.

Clinical History

A 28-year-old female with intractable temporal lobe seizures.

Findings

The dual echo coronal T2-weighted sequences (77A, 77B) demonstrate a subtle alteration of signal intensity within the posterior hippocampus of the left temporal lobe. This is seen as elevation of signal intensity on both sequences. The T1-weighted axial study (77C) demonstrates a small focal cystic collection in the white matter just beneath the parahippocampal gyrus, in the same region (77C, arrow). Note that a scan obtained five years earlier (77D) at a lower field strength demonstrates the same findings. There is no obvious mass effect. No vasogenic edema is seen in the adjacent white matter. An angiogram was done and was negative.

Diagnosis

Mesial temporal sclerosis.

Discussion

The surgical series in patients with intractable temporal lobe "partial complex" seizures have shown mesial temporal gliosis in the vast majority. However, in up to 28% of the cases, macroscopic structural lesions can be seen. These include tumors, as well as occult arteriovenous malformations. In true mesial temporal sclerosis, MR demonstrates T2-weighted signal abnormalities that correlate with the epileptogenic focus in only 8% of the cases. A major clue to such a benign entity is the presence of temporal horn enlargement associated with the temporal lesion, indicating some atrophy. In this particular case, the cystic change within the posterior hippocampus suggests the same entity; however, pathologic proof is lacking. Nevertheless, the five year interval between scans and the lack of any progression on the images strongly favor the benign entity as does the cystic change. However, because very slowly growing astrocytomas can occur in this location, that entity is not completely excluded despite the long interval of follow up.

References

1. Brooks BS, King DW, El Gammal T, et al. MR imaging in patients with intractable complex partial epileptic seizures. *AJNR* 1990;11:93–99.
2. Laster DW, Perry JK, Moody DM, et al. Chronic seizure disorders: contribution of MR when CT is normal. *AJNR* 1985;6:177–180.

Submitted by: Michael Brant-Zawadzki, M.D., Senior Editor.

163

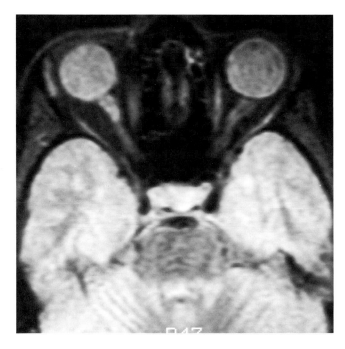

FIG. 78A. IR 2,000/30/130.

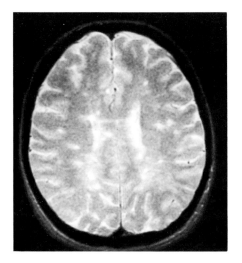

FIG. 78B. SE 2,800/70.

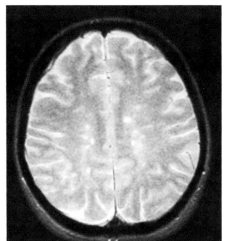

FIG. 78C. SE 2,800/70.

Clinical History

A 48-year-old female with acute loss of vision in the right eye. No significant prior history.

Findings

Short TI-inversion recovery image of the orbital mid-plane section (78A) reveals elevated signal intensity in the distal right optic nerve. Note the absence of signal from the orbital fat produced by the short TI-inversion recovery technique (SE 2,000/30, TI 130, 1.5T). The routine spin-echo (second echo) T2-weighted image at a higher level shows multiple foci of abnormality in the white matter typical of small MS plaques (78B, 78C).

Diagnosis

Optic neuritis associated with multiple sclerosis.

Discussion

Isolated idiopathic optic neuritis without clinical evidence of other central nervous system lesions may be the first manifestation of multiple sclerosis. Recent studies have shown that, with the use of MRI, one can detect silent MS plaques in the white matter of patients who present with isolated optic neuritis. In fact, one recent study suggests that up to half of the patients who experience an episode of idiopathic optic neuritis will harbor one or more lesions of the brain that are clinically silent but are revealed on MRI.

The inversion recovery technique has been studied with some depth in terms of its ability to highlight lesions in the white matter and optic nerves. Conventional T2-weighted spin-echo sequences best define lesions in the brain; however, the advantage of the short TI-inversion recovery technique in suppressing the high signal of fat in the orbits is obvious here. Other fat suppression techniques may help in this region as well.

References

1. Jacobs L, Kinkel PR, Kinkel WR. Silent brain lesions in patients with isolated idiopathic optic neuritis. *Arch Neurol* 1983;43:452–454.
2. Rung VM, Price AC, Kirshner HS, et al. Magnetic resonance imaging of multiple sclerosis: a study of pulse technique efficacy. *AJNR* 1984;5:691–702.

Submitted by: Michael Brant-Zawadzki, M.D., Senior Editor.

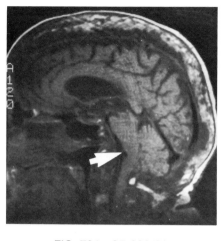

FIG. 79A. SE 600/20.

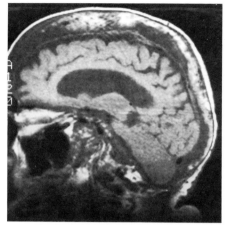

FIG. 79B. SE 600/20.

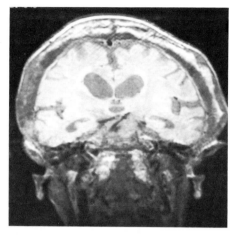

FIG. 79C. SE 2,000/20.

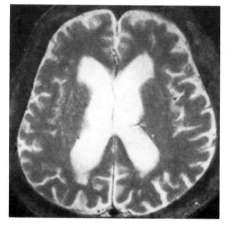

FIG. 79D. SE 2,800/80.

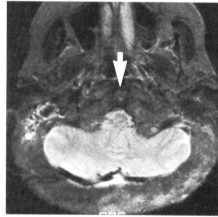

FIG. 79E. SE 2,800/80.

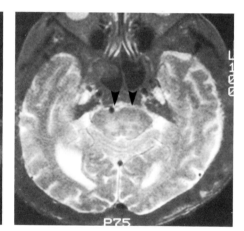

FIG. 79F. SE 2,800/80.

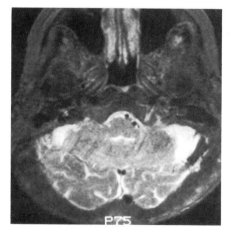

FIG. 79G. SE 2,800/80.

Clinical History

A 76-year-old woman with known Paget's disease presents with incontinence, dizziness, and swallowing difficulties.

Findings

The 5 mm axial T2-W (SE 2,800/80), 5 mm coronal (SE 2,000/20), and 5 mm sagittal (SE 600/20) images are presented.

There is extensive thickening of the calvarium consistent with the diagnosis of Paget's disease (79A–79E). Marked basilar invagination results in a high position of the odontoid with respect to the skull base. The odontoid is not well seen on the T1 sagittal images (79A), presumably due to involvement with Paget's disease, but it can be seen on the axial image (79E, white arrow). There is resulting deformity of the brainstem with compression of the inferior pons (79F, arrowheads) and abnormal angulation at the pontomedullary junction (79A, white arrow). There is also a narrowing of the 4th ventricle (79G). The cerebellar hemispheres are abnormally shaped (79B), particularly posteroinferiorly, and there is compression anteroinferiorly in the region of the flocculi bilaterally (79E). There is dilatation of the 3rd and lateral ventricular system out of proportion to the degree of dilatation of the basal cisterns and cerebral sulci (79D). There is no evidence of a smooth rim of increased signal in the periventricular region.

Patchy regions of increased signal intensity are present bilaterally in the pons, more marked on the right side (79F), and there are bilateral punctate foci of increased signal intensity in the deep white matter bilaterally.

Diagnosis

Paget's disease with basilar impression, brainstem compression and resultant compensated obstructive hydrocephalus; small brainstem infarcts and deep white matter infarcts.

Discussion

Basilar invagination in this case has occurred secondary to the bone-softening processes affecting the skull base. It occurs in approximately one-third of patients with Paget's disease of the skull, in the osteosclerotic phase, and with an increased frequency in severe disease and in females. Clinical findings of brainstem or upper cervical cord compression and cranial nerve dysfunction may occur, and there may be sufficient distortion to produce an obstructive hydrocephalus. In this case, the obstructive hydrocephalus occurs at the level of the aqueduct, likely due to brainstem distortion. The hydrocephalus is compensated, evidenced by a lack of the smooth margin of periventricular high signal seen in more acute cases.

Reference

1. Roberts MC, Kressel HY, Fellon MD, et al. Paget's disease: MR imaging findings. *Radiology* 1989;173:341–345.

Submitted by: Stephen J. Davis, M.D. and Louis M. Teresi, M.D., Huntington Medical Research Institutes, Pasadena, California; William G. Bradley, Jr., M.D., Ph.D., Senior Editor.

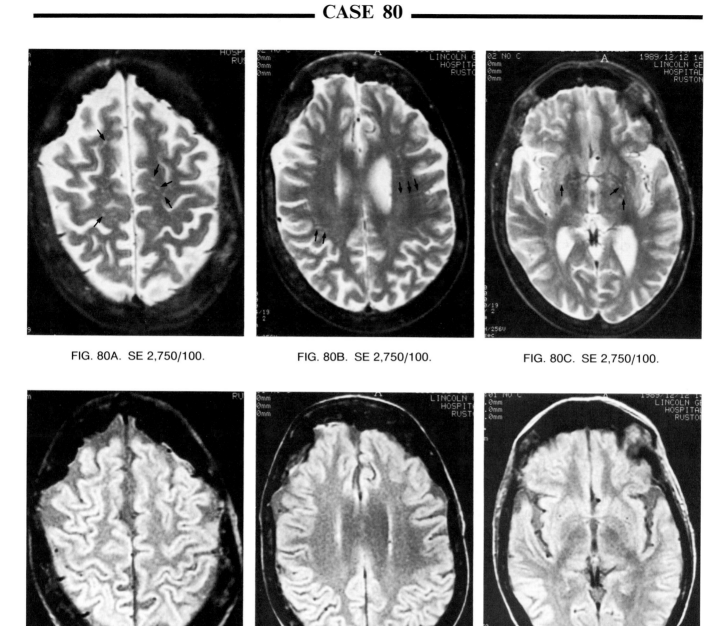

FIG. 80A. SE 2,750/100.

FIG. 80B. SE 2,750/100.

FIG. 80C. SE 2,750/100.

FIG. 80D. SE 2,750/25.

FIG. 80E. SE 2,750/25.

FIG. 80F. SE 2,750/25.

Clinical History

A 71-year-old female with headaches.

Findings

Axial 5 mm T2-W (SE 2,750/25 and 100) images are presented.

There are punctate foci of increased signal intensity in the subcortical region overlying the vertex of both cerebral hemispheres (80A). These punctate foci are best seen on the second echo of the T2-weighted sequence and are not well visualized on the first echo (80D). Multiple linear bands of increased signal with similar signal characteristics are also seen radiating from the periven-tricular white matter adjacent to the superior aspect of the lateral ventricles (80B, black arrows). Again, these are not visible on the first echo of the long TR sequence (80E). Similar intensity punctate foci are seen adjacent to the anterior commisure (80C, black arrows; 80F).

There is diffuse prominence of the cortical sulci bilaterally and mild prominence of the cerebellar sulci. Thickening of the inner table of the calvarium is noted bilaterally in the frontal region (80B).

Diagnosis

Prominent Virchow-Robin (perivascular) spaces; cortical atrophy; mild hyperostosis frontalis interna.

Discussion

The Virchow-Robin (perivascular) spaces are extensions of the subarachnoid space around the penetrating arteries, seen to the level of the capillaries, containing CSF. They are commonly seen adjacent to the anterior commissure in the inferior third of the basal ganglia where the lenticulostriate arteries enter the basal ganglia through the anterior perforated substance. They are also seen in the high convexity gray matter, extending inferiorly into the centrum semiovale following the course of penetrating cortical arterioles. They are of importance in that they need to be differentiated from white matter infarcts and basal ganglia lacunes. The signal intensity of perivascular spaces follows that of CSF, and therefore the "lesions" are not visible on moderately T2-weighted sequences, i.e., those in which CSF and brain are isointense. Such is the case on the first echo of the long TR sequence shown here (SE 2,750/25) at .5 T.

Simple enlargement of the perivascular spaces must be differentiated from *état criblé*, or cribiform atrophy, in which dilated perivascular spaces may be seen in combination with a narrow border of gliosis and/or perivascular demyelination (atrophic perivascular demyelination). In these cases, the abnormal brain tissue surrounding the dilated perivascular spaces may have increased signal intensity on moderately T2-weighted sequences.

Basal ganglia lacunes may be difficult to differentiate from enlarged perivascular spaces, but lacunes typically involve the upper two-thirds of the basal ganglia and do not follow CSF intensity on all sequences. They also tend to be less symmetrical than perivascular spaces. Although large Virchow-Robin spaces are associated with hypertension, dementia, and incidental white matter lesions, this association is thought to be due to the aging process rather than its representing an independent association.

Hyperostosis frontalis interna occurs in up to 8% of elderly women. Fatty marrow within the bones may occasionally simulate subdural collections on T1-weighted images.

References

1. Drayer BP. Imaging of the aging brain, Parts I and II. *Radiology* 1988;166:785–806.
2. Heier LA, Bauer CJ, Schwartz L, et al. Large Virchow-Robin spaces: MR-clinical correlation. *AJNR* 1989;10:929–936.

Submitted by: Stephen J. Davis, M.D. and Louis M. Teresi, M.D., Huntington Medical Research Institutes, Pasadena, California; William G. Bradley, Jr., M.D., Ph.D., Senior Editor.

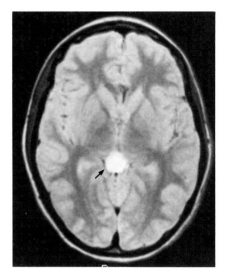

FIG. 81A. SE 3,000/40.

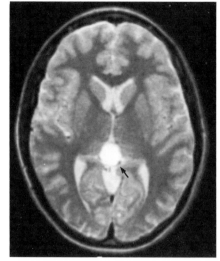

FIG. 81B. SE 3,000/80.

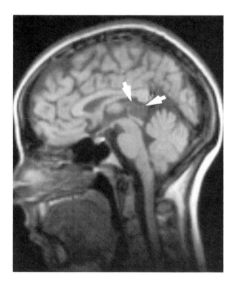

FIG. 81C. SE 500/40.

Clinical History

A 20-year-old woman with headaches.

Findings

Axial 5 mm T2-W (SE 3,000/40 and 80) and sagittal 5 mm T1-W (SE 500/40) images are presented.

There is a homogeneous, well-defined mass measuring 1.7 cm in diameter in the pineal region. The mass is rounded, circumscribed, and sharply marginated, and it has a homogeneous internal signal showing increased signal intensity on both the first and second echo of the T2-weighted images (81A, 81B), and slight increase in signal intensity on the T1-weighted images when compared to surrounding CSF (81C). The lesion separates the internal cerebral veins (81A, 81B, black arrows) and is mildly indented superiorly by the splenium of the corpus callosum (81C). There is mild impression upon the tectum of the midbrain, but there is no evidence of obstruction of the cerebral aqueduct. There is no evidence of calcification or hemorrhage.

Diagnosis

Benign pineal cyst.

Discussion

Pineal cysts occurred in 4.3% of one large series of patients. The pineal gland arises from a diverticulum of the 3rd ventricle that, while closing off, commonly gives rise to small cavities within the gland that are lined by primitive cells capable of differentiating into ependyma or neuroglia. Those with ependymal lining may go on to become large cysts. These cysts need to be differentiated from more significant pineal tumors. Cysts are characteristically slightly more intense than CSF on T1-weighted images and much more intense than CSF on T2-weighted images, as shown in this case. This is due to elevated protein content of the cyst fluid, causing mild T1 shortening when compared to the adjacent CSF. On the T2-weighted image, the cyst appears brighter than CSF because of predominance of this T1 effect. Pineal cysts under 1.5 cm in diameter can be categorically diagnosed by MR. Larger pineal cysts can cause hydrocephalus from aqueductal obstruction. Large pineal cysts should undergo CT scanning to exclude calcification and to confirm the diagnosis of benignancy. Larger cysts should also be scanned with contrast by either CT or MR as central enhancement suggests tumor. Mild peripheral enhancement can be seen in benign cysts, however. In contrast to pineal cysts, pineal tumors, as well as showing a shorter T2 (due to the more solid components). They may present with mass effect leading to Parinaud's syndrome (failure of upgaze) due to tectal compression, diplopia, headache, and obstructive hydrocephalus.

Reference

1. Mamourian AC, Towfighi J. Pineal cysts: MR imaging. *AJNR* 1986;7:1081–1086.

Submitted by: Stephen J. Davis, M.D. and Louis M. Teresi, M.D., Huntington Medical Research Institutes, Pasadena, California; William G. Bradley, Jr., M.D., Ph.D., Senior Editor.

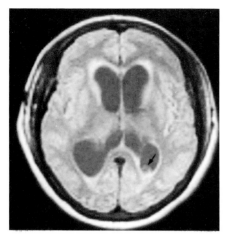

FIG. 82A. SE 2,000/28.

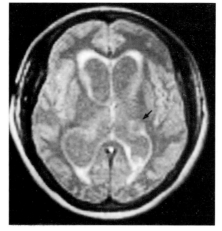

FIG. 82B. SE 2,000/56.

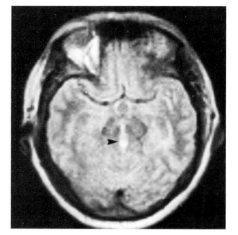

FIG. 82C. SE 2,000/56.

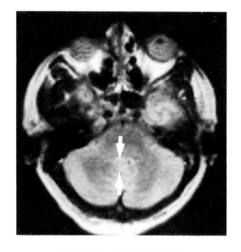

FIG. 82D. SE 2,000/56.

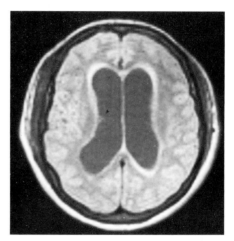

FIG. 82E. SE 2,000/28.

Clinical History

A 50-year-old woman with a two-month history of headaches and vomiting.

Findings

Axial 7 mm T2-W (SE 2,000/28 and 56) images are presented. There is generalized enlargement of the 3rd and lateral ventricles. A thin, smooth border of high intensity surrounds the lateral ventricles (82B, 82E). There are two 1 cm in diameter thin-rimmed cystic structures adjacent to the ventricular wall in the posterior horn of the left lateral ventricle (82A, 82B, black arrows). The anterior cystic lesion appears to arise within the ventricular wall, whereas the more posterior lesion is more intraventricular.

There is a 5 mm high-intensity lesion within the proximal cerebral aqueduct (82C, arrowhead). A further 1 cm rounded lesion is noted, distorting the right side of the 4th ventricle (82D, white arrows). This latter lesion has an appearance similar to the two cystic lesions in the posterior horn of the left lateral ventricle. A 5 mm lesion arises from the lateral aspect of the body of the right lateral ventricle (82E, black arrowhead). A 2 cm diameter mucous retention cyst in the inferior left maxillary sinus is incidentally noted.

Diagnosis

Intraventricular cysticercosis with acute obstructive hydrocephalus at the level of the aqueduct.

Discussion

Neurocysticercosis is an infection of the CNS by the larval form of the pork tapeworm *Taenia solium*. The ingested ova release the larval form in the stomach, penetrate the intestinal mucosa, and then have a predilection for localizing in skin, muscle, and the CNS where they typically involve the cerebral gray matter, periventricular tissues, or leptomeninges. The larval cells proliferate, producing 1–2 cm diameter cysts. The parasite may die, resulting in cyst degeneration and a striking host inflammatory response and gliotic reaction.

Intraventricular cysts are generally isointense relative to CSF, as in this case, although the intracyst fluid may show a slightly increased intensity relative to CSF, possibly related to cyst degeneration or lack of flow. A pericystic ependymal inflammatory reaction is common. Intraventricular cysts may remain clinically silent until they degenerate, causing an ependymal reaction, or until they cause obstructive hydrocephalus.

Treatment with praziquantel can result in resolution of intraventricular cysts.

Reference

1. Teitelbaum G, Otto RJ, Lin M, et al. MR imaging of neurocysticercosis. *AJNR* 1989;10:709–718.

Submitted by: Stephen J. Davis, M.D. and Louis M. Teresi, M.D., Huntington Medical Research Institutes, Pasadena, California; William G. Bradley, Jr., M.D., Ph.D., Senior Editor.

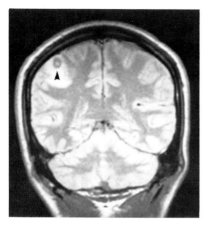

FIG. 83A. SE 2,500/22.

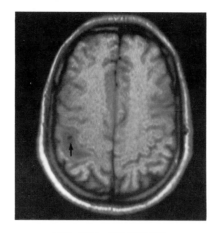

FIG. 83B. SE 850/20.

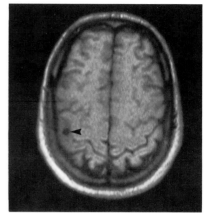

FIG. 83C. SE 850/20.

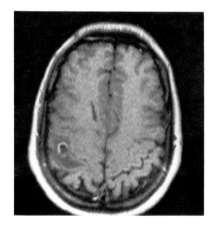

FIG. 83D. SE 850/20 with Gd-DPTA.

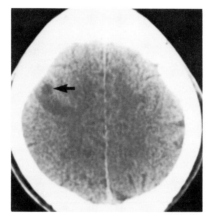

FIG. 83E. CT.

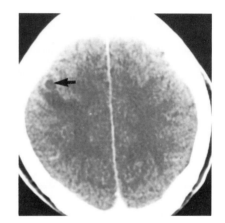

FIG. 83F. CT with contrast.

Clinical History

A 34-year-old Mexican immigrant with recent onset of seizures.

Findings

Axial 6 mm T1-W pre- and post-gadolinium (SE 850/20) and coronal 6 mm T2-W (SE 2500/22 and 80) MR images and enhanced and unenhanced CT scans are presented.

There is a 1 cm diameter cystic lesion situated at the gray-white interface of the superolateral aspect of the right parietal lobe (83A, 83C, black arrowheads). The signal intensity within the cyst follows that of CSF on both T1- and T2-weighted sequences. In addition, within the cyst there is a focus of increased signal (83A, 83B, small black arrows). Surrounding the lesion and extending into the adjacent white matter is a 3 cm irregularly marginated region of increased signal intensity on the T2-weighted images, with corresponding low signal intensity on the T1-weighted images. There is mild associated mass effect with effacement of the adjacent cerebral sulci.

Diagnosis

Parenchymal neurocysticercosis.

Discussion

The features of an isolated cysticercosis cyst are classical. These lesions typically locate at the gray-white interface and are usually 1–2 cm in diameter, although lesions up to 4 cm in size have been reported. The cysts survive for approximately five years before they degenerate. During this time, the internal signal characteristics of the cyst parallel the intensity of CSF in multiple sequences. The focal intracystic high signal (83A, 83B, black arrows) represents the scolex, which can be recognized in approximately 50% of cysts.

With the death of the cysticercosis larvae, the cyst degenerates, producing higher signal intensity within the cyst when compared to the CSF on T1-weighted and long TR/short TE sequences. Pericystic edema and gliosis are also more pronounced with degenerating cysts. Although there is pronounced pericystic edema, or gliosis, in this case, the internal characteristics of the cyst on MR and the lack of calcification on noncontrast CT (83E) suggests that the cyst is still likely to be viable. Rim enhancement of the cyst wall with gadolinium (83D) and with iodine in the post-contrast CT (83F, arrow) is noted. Lack of pericystic contrast enhancement (rather than cystic wall enhancement) also favors a viable rather than a degenerative cyst.

Reference

1. Teitelbaum GP, Otto RJ, Lin M, et al. MR imaging of neurocysticercosis. *AJNR* 1989;10:709–718. (See also Case 82 on intraventricular cysticercosis.)

Submitted by: Stephen J. Davis, M.D. and Louis M. Teresi, M.D., Huntington Medical Research Institutes, Pasadena, California; William G. Bradley, Jr., M.D., Ph.D., Senior Editor.

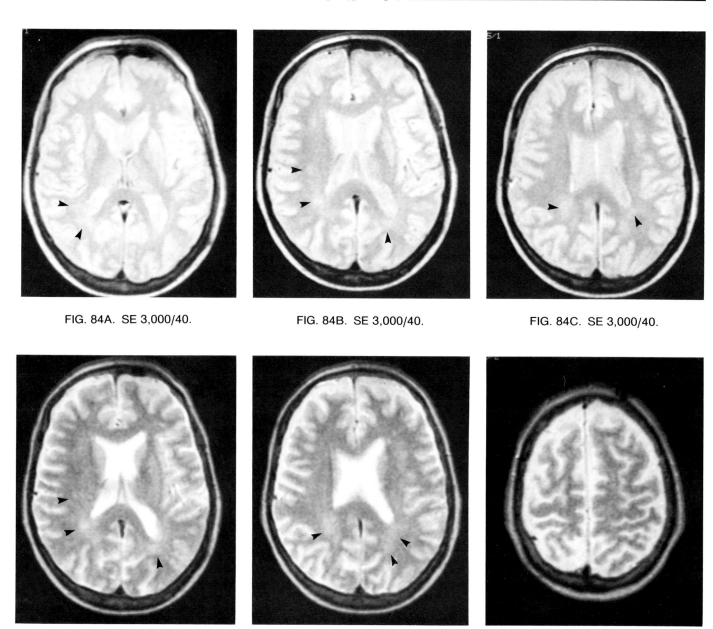

FIG. 84A. SE 3,000/40.

FIG. 84B. SE 3,000/40.

FIG. 84C. SE 3,000/40.

FIG. 84D. SE 3,000/80.

FIG. 84E. SE 3,000/80.

FIG. 84F. SE 3,000/80.

Clinical History

A 68-year-old severe hemophiliac with depression.

Findings

Axial 5 mm T2-W (SE 3,000/40 and 80) images are presented. There are diffuse areas of increased signal intensity throughout the deep white matter, particularly involving the major forceps (84A–84E, black arrowheads). The ventricles and cortical sulci are mildly prominent (84F).

Diagnosis

"Dirty white matter" and mild cortical atrophy consistent with human immunodeficiency virus (HIV) encephalitis.

Discussion

Approximately 30% of patients with HIV infection have MR evidence of white matter disease. In most cases, the white matter abnormalities are seen in patients with the AIDS dementia complex (ADC), caused by direct infection of glial cells with the HIV. The most common MR pattern observed in patients with ADC is that of diffuse high signal intensity in the periventricular white matter on T2-weighted images. Patchy or punctate white matter lesions may also be seen, but these are not as common. Focal, well-defined areas of white matter disease are also seen in patients with progressive multifocal leukoencephalopathy (PML) and occasionally in toxoplasmosis or lymphoma. If a focal white matter lesion is identified with MR imaging, gadolinium enhancement is advised, since toxoplasmosis and lymphoma usually enhance whereas PML almost never does.

This patient's white matter lesions are best classified as "patchy," being localized lesions with ill-defined margins. Although the diffuse white matter pattern is the most common pattern in patients with ADC, patchy changes, as in this case, are the next most frequent finding. Clinical features are also useful in distinguishing ADC from other causes of white matter disease. ADC patients rarely have focal neurological findings whereas these are common with PML. Patchy white matter disease is found in a variety of clinical settings, including ADC, Cryptococcus meningitis, and suspected toxoplasmosis.

References

1. Olsen WL, Longo FM, Mills CM, Norman D. White matter disease in AIDS: Findings at MR imaging. *Radiology* 1988;169:445–448.
2. Sze G, Brant-Zawadzki MN, Norman D, et al. Neuroradiology of AIDS. *Semin Roentgenol* 1987;22:42.

Submitted by: Stephen J. Davis, M.D. and Louis M. Teresi, M.D., Huntington Medical Research Institutes, Pasadena, California; William G. Bradley, Jr., M.D., Ph.D., Senior Editor.

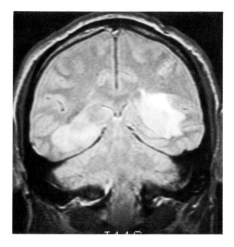

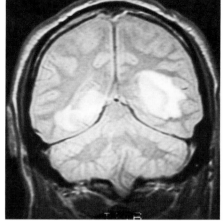

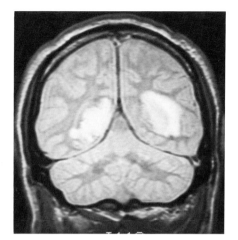

FIG. 85A. SE 2,800/30.   FIG. 85B. SE 2,800/30.   FIG. 85C. SE 2,800/30.

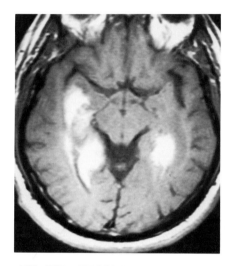

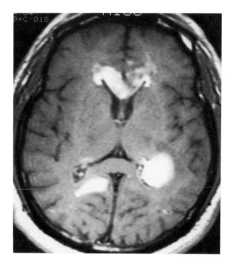

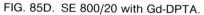

FIG. 85D. SE 800/20 with Gd-DPTA.   FIG. 85E. SE 800/20 with Gd-DPTA.

Clinical History

A 60-year-old male with recent memory loss and progressive confusion.

Findings

The T2-weighted images show subependymal lesion spread on the coronal images (85A–85C). Following paramagnetic contrast injection, the axial images show the diffuse nature of the subependymal process. A homogeneously enhancing plate of tissue surrounds the perimeter of the ventricular system, with lobulation of the lesion margins (85D, 85E).

Diagnosis

Primary lymphoma.

Discussion

Systemic lymphoma can spread to the brain from any primary focus. Most often, this is an immunoblastic form of lymphoma (formally known as *diffuse histiocytic lymphoma*). Most typically, such secondary brain involvement by lymphoma is in the meninges, with CSF sampling being the diagnostic modality used to detect it. Such spread occurs through cranial nerves centrally. However, hematogenous spread of lymphoma to the brain can also occur, producing mass lesions. The lesions tend to be homogeneous in appearance, with relatively little edema. Hodgkin's disease rarely involves the brain. When seen, it often affects the dura.

Primary brain lymphoma was formerly called micro-glioma. Typical location is in the subependymal region, either as a single mass lesion or with subependymal spread. Occasionally, a magnetically susceptible effect within the lymphomatous lesion can be seen as an area of lowered signal intensity. Hemorrhage within lymphoma is quite uncommon.

The differential diagnosis of diffuse subependymal spread of disease includes primary brain tumors, such as glioma, medulloblastoma, and ependymoma, as well as metastatic tumor (typically adenocarcinoma). Chronic infections can occasionally produce this appearance. Interstitial edema from hydrocephalus generally shows a thinner rim with no lobulation (and would not enhance).

References

1. Jack C et al. Radiographic findings in 32 cases of primary CNS lymphoma. *AJNR* 1985;6:899–904.
2. Davis P et al. Leptomeningeal metastasis: MR imaging. *Radiology* 1987;163:449–454.
3. Brant-Zawadzki MN et al. Primary intracranial tumor imaging: a comparison of magnetic resonance and CT. *Radiology* 1984;150:435–438.
4. Graif C et al. Contrast enhanced MR imaging of malignant brain tumors. *AJNR* 1985;6:855–862.
5. Kilgore D et al. Cranial tissues: normal MR appearance after intravenous injection of Gd-DTPA. *Radiology* 1986;160:757–761.

Submitted by: Michael Brant-Zawadzki, M.D., Senior Editor.

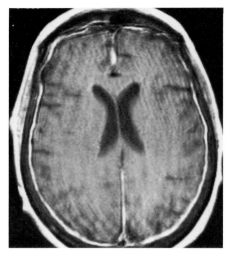 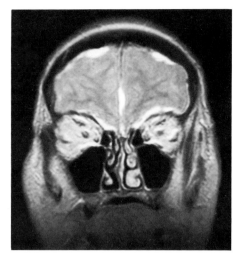

FIG. 86A. SE 800/20 with Gd-DPTA.   FIG. 86B. SE 800/20 with Gd-DPTA.

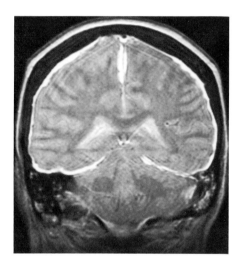

FIG. 86C. SE 2,800/30 with Gd-DPTA.

Clinical History

A 74-year-old female with known CNS spread of immunoblastic systemic lymphoma status post intrathecal chemotherapy treatment, altered consciousness.

Findings

The T1-weighted axial image (86A) following intravenous paramagnetic contrast administration shows a relatively symmetric-appearing enhancement of the dura. Note that the enhancement of the dura extends into the inner hemispheric region corresponding to the falx (the remainder of the intrahemispheric fissure, the sulci, do not show enhancement). However, the coronal first echo, T2-weighted sequences (86B, 86C) show that the enhancement of the dura is rather lobulated and irregular in appearance. Note that the falx can be seen as a thin linear low signal stripe within the midst of the enhancing dural space. Also, the dural abnormality extends to the tentorial roof.

Diagnosis

Immunoblastic lymphoma.

Discussion

Enhancement of the dura is problematic. Any generalized insult will produce a reaction of the dura—thickening and hypervascularity of the membrane occurs. Thus, with trauma, irritation due to ventricular shunt placement, prior hemorrhage, or surgery can all produce nonspecific dural enhancement. This should be smooth and regular in appearance, as in the axial T1-weighted image of this case. However, spread of tumor to the dura can also occur. Once lobulation of the dural thickening is seen (the type of irregularity shown on the coronal sequences here), tumor involvement must be suspected. Contrast enhancement is vital to the demonstration of subtle leptomeningeal or dural pathology.

References

1. Jack C et al. Radiographic findings in 32 cases of primary CNS lymphoma. *AJNR* 1985;6:899–904.
2. Davis P et al. Leptomeningeal metastasis: MR imaging. *Radiology* 1987;163:449–454.
3. Brant-Zawadzki MN et al. Primary intracranial tumor imaging: a comparison of magnetic resonance and CT. *Radiology* 1984;150:435–438.
4. Graif C et al. Contrast enhanced MR imaging of malignant brain tumors. *AJNR* 1985;6:855–862.
5. Kilgore D et al. Cranial tissues: normal MR appearance after intravenous injection of Gd-DTPA. *Radiology* 1986;160:757–761.

Submitted by: Michael Brant-Zawadzki, M.D., Senior Editor.

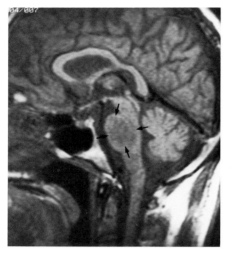

FIG. 87A. SE 500/20.

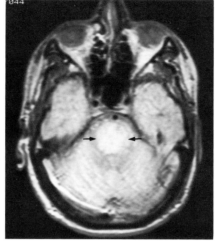

FIG. 87B. SE 2,500/35.

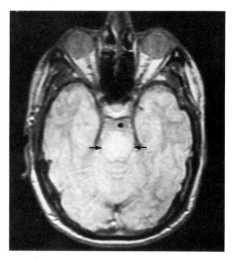

FIG. 87C. SE 2,500/35.

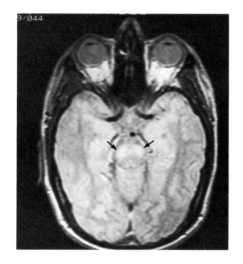

FIG. 87D. SE 2,500/35.

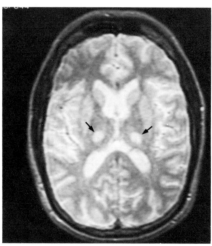

FIG. 87E. SE 2,500/70.

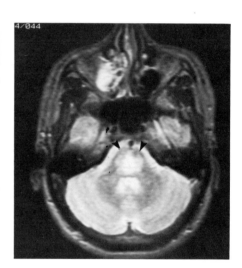

FIG. 87F. SE 2,500/70.

Clinical History

A 34-year-old male with a 15-year history of alcohol abuse presented one month prior to this scan with mental obtundation, quadriparesis, and severe electrolyte imbalance with hyponatremia. The quadriparesis had almost completely resolved at the time of this scan.

Findings

Axial 5 mm T2-W (SE 2,500/35 and 70) and sagittal 5 mm T1-W (SE 500/20) images are presented.

There is a large, fairly discrete lesion measuring approximately 2.5 cm involving almost the entire basis pontis with sparing only of a thin rim of tissue anteriorly and the pontine tegmentum posteriorly. This shows decreased signal intensity on T1-weighted images (87A, arrows) and increased signal on T2-weighted sequences (87B, 87C, 87D, arrows). The lesion extends superiorly to end just inferior to the red nuclei and substantia nigra of the midbrain, and inferiorly to the pontomedullary junction. There are scattered punctate foci of similar sig-nal change in the upper medulla. Despite the size of the pontine lesion, there is no evidence of mass effect or obstruction of the aqueduct.

There are bilateral symmetrical 1 cm oval lesions similar to the pontine lesion, involving the dorsal and lateral nuclei of the thalami bilaterally (87E).

There are also scattered punctate foci of increased signal intensity in the periventricular white matter bilaterally, consistent with mild, deep white matter ischemic changes. There is also complete opacification of the right maxillary sinus with mucoperiosteal thickening of the right middle and anterior ethmoidal sinuses.

Diagnosis

Central pontine myelinolysis; extrapontine myelinolysis involving the thalami bilaterally.

Discussion

Central pontine myelinolysis is characterized by regions of demyelination throughout the brain that are most prominent in the pons. The lesions are characteristically found in chronic alcoholics with hyponatremia, although they may be seen in any patient in which hyponatremia has been corrected rapidly. These patients present with an acute illness characterized by spastic quadriparesis, pseudobulbar palsy, and mental obtundation. Although many patients die, survival with varying neurological residua (including a relatively mild sequella as in this patient) is increasingly recognized. Pathologically, symmetrical demyelination at the base of the pons spreading from the median raphe is characteristic with relative sparing of the ventrolateral longitudinal fibers. In severe cases, there is necrosis and cavitation as well as extension into the pontine tegmentum and midbrain. Symmetrical foci in other parts of the brain, including the basal ganglia, thalami, cerebral peduncles, corticomedullary junctions of the cerebrum and cerebellum, and spinal cord have also been documented.

The most common finding is symmetric round or oval areas of prolonged T1 and T2 within the base of the pons. There is usually sparing of the ventrolateral aspect of the pons (87F, arrowheads) that may result in a trident-shaped lesion in axial images. In all cases, the peripheral portion of the pons is spared. The extrapontine sites shown in this case show the typical symmetrical appearance in a characteristic site (thalami). The initial MR images may appear normal, particularly within one week of symptom onset. One to two weeks later the lesion may appear quite large, involving nearly the entire pons, due to demyelination and edema, but as time progresses the lesion becomes smaller and better defined and more accurately reflects the degree of demyelination. Absence of obstructive hydrocephalus and the clinical presentation are strongly in favor of central pontine myelinolysis, but the MR features are not specific. Other demyelinating diseases, gliomas, and leukoencephalopathies may have similar appearances, although in the latter, the supratentorial white matter disease is usually much more prominent.

Reference

1. Miller GM, Baker HL, Okazaki H, Whisnant JP. Central pontine myelinolysis and its imitators: MR findings. *Radiology* 1988;168:795–802.

Submitted by: Stephen J. Davis, M.D. and Louis M. Teresi, M.D., Huntington Medical Research Institutes, Pasadena, California; William G. Bradley, Jr., M.D., Ph.D., Senior Editor.

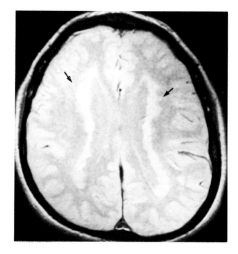

FIG. 88A. SE 2,800/30.

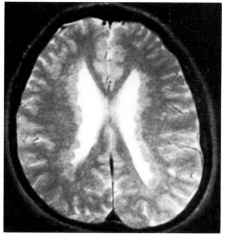

FIG. 88B. SE 2,800/80.

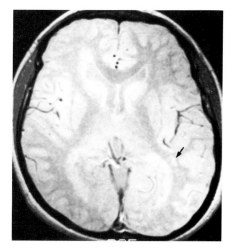

FIG. 88C. SE 2,800/30.

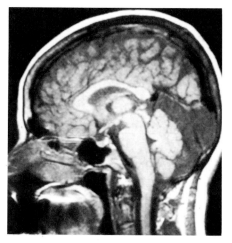

FIG. 88D. SE 600/20.

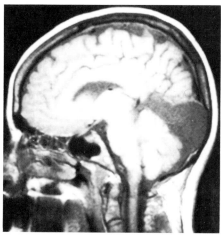

FIG. 88E. SE 600/20.

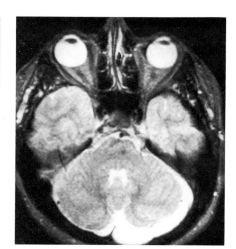

FIG. 88F. SE 2,800/80.

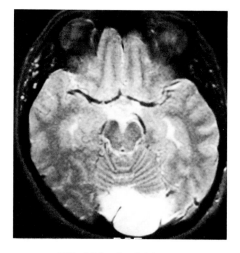

FIG. 88G. SE 2,800/80.

Clinical History

A 45-year-old female with long-standing convulsive disorder.

Findings

Axial 5 mm T2-W (SE 2,000/30 and 80) and sagittal 5 mm T1-W (SE 600/20) images are presented.

There is nodular irregularity of the lateral walls of both lateral ventricles. This is caused by an irregular 1 cm band of tissue surrounding the lateral ventricles that has the same signal intensity as gray matter (88A, 88B).

There are multiple small nodules in the deep white matter (88A, 88C, black arrows). These nodules similarly follow the signal intensity of gray matter and are not well seen on the second echo (88B).

There is a CSF intensity collection in the midline in the posterior fossa (88D, 88E, 88G). This collection is more prominent to the left of midline (88G) and displaces the falx cerebelli to the right, the posterior tentorium superiorly (88E), and erodes the inner table of the occiput (88E). The cerebellar vermis is well formed (88F), and no cerebellar hypoplasia or other malformation is evident.

Diagnosis

Heterotopic gray matter; posterior fossa arachnoid cyst.

Discussion

Heterotopic gray matter results from failure of neuroepithelial cells to migrate from the periventricular germinal matrix to the cortical surface. Migrational failures can result in polymicrogyria with an increased number of smaller-than-normal gyri, pacchygyria, characterized by a few broad gyri separated by decreased number of sulci or its extreme form, lissencephaly, where there is little or no cortical gyration. The lack of migration produces nests of periventricular cells that project into the ventricle. There is no gliosis associated with this process, and the tissue therefore has the same signal intensity as normal gray matter. It should be differentiated from subependymal nodules of tuberous sclerosis that are often calcified and associated with other characteristic abnormalities.

Heterotopic gray matter may occur anywhere from the ependymal lining of the ventricle to the cortex. There are several such small nodules in this patient, measuring 2–4 mm in diameter (88A, 88C, black arrows). Of note is the fact that, although they have a mild increase in signal intensity with respect to the deep white matter on the first echo of the T2-weighted sequence, they do not show an increase in signal intensity on the second echo and, instead, follow the signal intensity of gray matter. These should not be confused with deep white matter infarcts or multiple sclerotic plaques. Heterotopias may be asymptomatic, although, if there is extensive involvement, they may present with seizures or mental retardation.

Discrete posterior fossa CSF collections that are clearly separate from the 4th ventricle and vallecula are classified as posterior fossa cysts, whereas those that communicate with the 4th ventricle and are associated with cerebellar atrophy are termed *prominent cisterna magna*. Both can cause enlargement of the posterior fossa and scalloping of the inner table of the occipital bone. In this case, the fact that there is no evidence of cerebellar malformation or hypoplasia and that the collection does not communicate with the 4th ventricle and vallecula make a diagnosis of arachnoid cyst most likely.

References

1. Barkovich AJ, Kjos BO, Norman D, Edwards MS. Revised classification of posterior fossa cysts and cystlike malformations based on the results of multiplanar MR imaging. *AJNR* 1990;10:977–988.
2. Hayden SA, Davis KA, Stears JC, et al. MR imaging of heterotopic grey matter. *JCAT* 1987;11:878.

Submitted by: Stephen J. Davis, M.D. and Louis M. Teresi, M.D., Huntington Medical Research Institutes, Pasadena, California; William G. Bradley, Jr., M.D., Ph.D., Senior Editor.

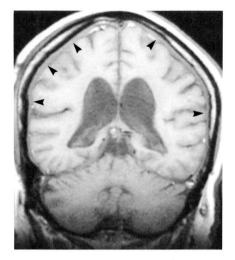

FIG. 89A. SE 500/20.

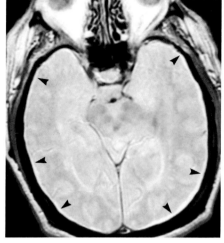

FIG. 89B. SE 3,000/30.

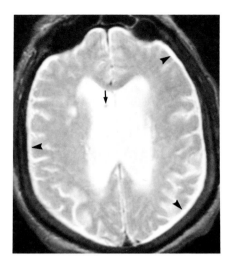

FIG. 89C. SE 3,000/80.

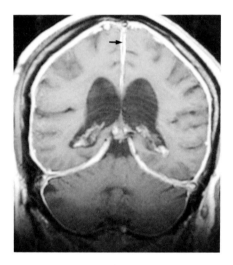

FIG. 89D. SE 500/20 with Gd-DPTA.

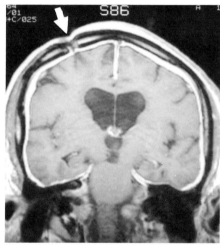

FIG. 89E. SE 500/20 with Gd-DPTA.

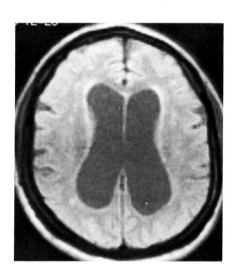

FIG. 89F. SE 2,000/28.

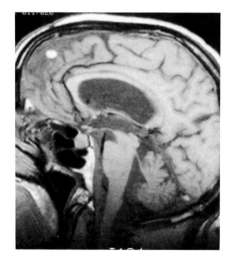

FIG. 89G. SE 500/20.

Clinical History

A 72-year-old male shunted for normal pressure hydrocephalus four years previously presents with blurring of left vision for three months for shunt assessment.

Findings

The 5 mm sagittal T1-W (SE 500/20), 5 mm coronal T1-W both pre- and post-gadolinium (SE 500/20), and axial 5 mm T2-W (SE 3,000/30 and 80) images are presented. Axial 10 mm (SE 2,000/28) images from four years previously, prior to shunting, are also presented.

There is a diffuse 3–5 mm rind of subdural tissue extending over both cerebral and cerebellar hemispheres following the subdural compartment into the interhemispheric fissue and along the tentorium (89A, 89B, 89C, arrowheads). This mantle is isointense with brain on T1-weighted images (89A) and hyperintense when compared to both CSF and brain on the first echo of the T2-weighted sequence (89B). Marked diffuse contrast enhancement of this mantle is shown, following gadolinium administration (89D, 89E), both in the supratentorial compartment where it is more marked and the infratentorial compartment. A ventricular shunt tube is noted in the right lateral ventricle (89C, black arrow) via a craniotomy defect in the right frontal bone (89E, white arrow). A very thin rim of high intensity signal is present around the dilated lateral ventricles, and the 3rd and 4th ventricles are also moderately enlarged. The ventricles show a slight decrease in size (89C) when compared to the pre-operative scan (89F). There are multiple focal areas of increased signal intensity in the periventricular white matter bilaterally.

There is a 1 cm diameter pituitary mass (89G). There is an 8 mm oval high intensity mass present adjacent to the falx anteriorly (89G).

Diagnosis

Benign meningeal fibrosis following placement of ventricular shunt; communicating hydrocephalus; deep white matter ischemic changes; pituitary tumor (asymptomatic); falx ossification.

Discussion

Benign meningeal fibrosis in the subdural space may occur following ventricular shunting. Although the cause of this fibrosis is unclear, it probably represents a complication of one or more subdural hemorrhages with neovascularization and fibrosis of the subdural space. It has also been reported in patients following subdural hematomas. These mimic the appearance of chronic thin subdural collections on unenhanced MR scans. However, following enhancement, a thick rind of enhancement is shown of the full thickness of the rind seen on the pre-contrast scan, clearly differentiating this fibrotic condition from a fluid collection. The normal falx and tentorium can be seen as thin dark lines (89D, black arrow) within the enhancing tissue. The clinical significance of this abnormality is uncertain. In addition to a previous operation, other causes of chemical meningitis, recurrent subarachnoid hemorrhage, or inflammatory meningitis may also give rise to benign meningeal enhancement.

The falx stone (89G) is a commonly seen normal variant and is due to ossification occurring in the falx. The intramedullary fat of the heterotopic ossification produces a bright signal on the T1 sequence, and this should not be confused with more significant pathology.

References

1. Destian S, Heier LA, Zimmerman RD, et al. Differentiation between meningeal fibrosis and chronic subdural hematoma after ventricular shunting: value of enhanced CT and MR scans. *AJNR* 1989;10:1021–1026.
2. Burke JW, Podrasky AL, Bradley WG. Meninges: benign postoperative enhancement on MR images. *Radiology* 1990;174:99–102.

Submitted by: Stephen J. Davis, M.D. and Louis M. Teresi, M.D., Huntington Medical Research Institutes, Pasadena, California; William G. Bradley, Jr., M.D., Ph.D., Senior Editor.

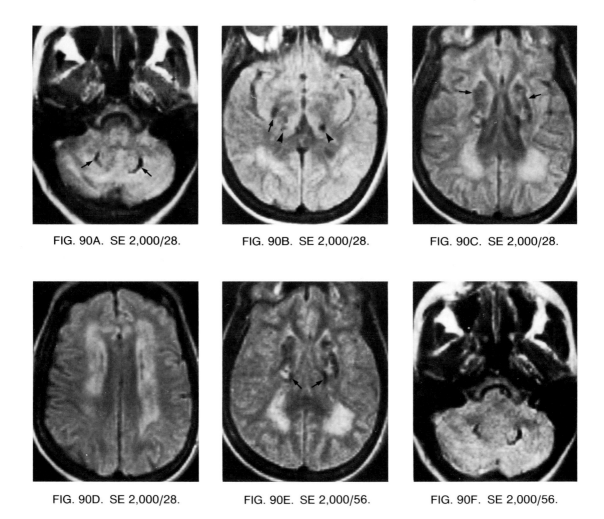

FIG. 90A. SE 2,000/28.   FIG. 90B. SE 2,000/28.   FIG. 90C. SE 2,000/28.

FIG. 90D. SE 2,000/28.   FIG. 90E. SE 2,000/56.   FIG. 90F. SE 2,000/56.

Clinical History

A 50-year-old woman with long-standing history of progressive movement disorder that began in adolescence.

Findings

Axial 7 mm T2-W (SE 2,000/28 and 56) images are presented.

There are multiple focal areas of reduced signal intensity involving the dentate nuclei (90A, arrows), the thalami (90B, arrowheads) with larger lesions bridging from the heads of the caudate nuclei to the putamen bilaterally (90B, 90C, arrows). The bodies of the caudate nuclei are also similarly involved (90E, arrows). These lesions do not show progressive signal loss between the first and second echos (compare 90C and 90E, and 90A and 90F) to indicate any selective T2 shortening.

There is confluent irregular increased signal intensity involving the white matter surrounding the lateral ventricles bilaterally (90C, 90D). There is no evidence of atrophy.

Diagnosis

Extensive basal ganglia calcification secondary to Fahr's disease.

Discussion

Calcification produces signal loss on all sequences. Although MR is not as sensitive or specific in the diagnosis of calcification as is CT, gradient echo techniques do provide greater sensitivity than do spin echoes. This is due to the gradient echo technique's intrinsic sensitivity to the magnetic susceptibility effect produced by calcium. The CT image (90G) shows more extensive calcification in the dentate nuclei than is demonstrated by the MR sequence. The regions of signal loss need to be differentiated from iron deposition that also typically occurs in the basal ganglia region in many conditions. For example, Hallervorden-Spatz disease also causes gradual development of progressive rigidity and an extrapyramidal movement disorder occurring over a period of years, as was seen in this case. Iron, however, shows greater T2 shortening, manifesting progressive loss of signal with lengthening of the TE. Iron shows less signal loss on T1-weighted sequences, which are less sensitive to susceptibility effects.

The causes of basal ganglia calcification include hypoparathyroidism, pseudohypoparathyroidism, and pseudo pseudohypoparathyroidism and idiopathic. Other causes include congenital cytomegalovirus (CMV) or toxoplasmosis infections, lead or carbon monoxide poisoning, tuberous sclerosis, Cockayne's syndrome, and Fahr's disease. In this case, hypoparathyroidism or pseudohypoparathyroidism would be compatible with the history and calcification but could be excluded by the absence of hypocalcemia. Fahr's syndrome has normal serum calcium.

References

1. Oot RF, New PJ, Pile-Spellman J, et al. The detection of intracranial calcifications by MR. *AJNR* 1986;7:801–809.
2. Tsuruda JS, Bradley WG, et al. MR detection of intracranial calcification: A phantom study. *AJNR* 1987;8:1049–1055.

Submitted by: Stephen J. Davis, M.D. and Louis M. Teresi, M.D., Huntington Medical Research Institutes, Pasadena, California; William G. Bradley, Jr., M.D., Ph.D., Senior Editor.

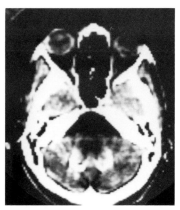

FIG. 90G. CT.

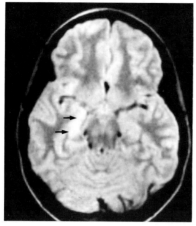 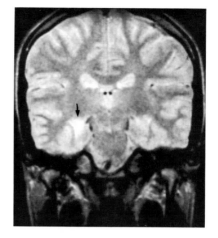

FIG. 91A. SE 3,000/40.   FIG. 91B. SE 2,000/80.

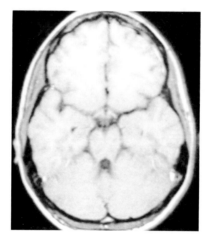

FIG. 91C. SE 500/30 with Gd-DPTA.

Clinical History

A 20-year-old female with long-standing temporal lobe epilepsy.

Findings

Axial 5 mm T2-W (SE 3,000/40), coronal 5 mm T2-W (SE 2,000/80), and post-gadolinium 5 mm T1-W (SE 500/30) images are presented.

There is ill-defined increased signal intensity involving the right hippocampal formation (91A, 91B, black arrows) when compared to the normal hippocampal formation on the left. There is no evidence of accompanying mass effect. Although atrophy is difficult to assess, the right temporal horn is larger than the left (91C). There was no evidence of gadolinium enhancement (91C).

Diagnosis

Probable mesial temporal sclerosis.

Discussion

In patients who finally undergo a temporal lobe resection for temporal lobe epilepsy, a specific morphological lesion is found in roughly 75%, with 25% of such cases showing grossly detectible lesions and the other 50% showing the pathological process to be hippocampal sclerosis, defined predominately by its microscopic appearance. Hippocampal sclerosis is characterized by selective neuronal necrosis with a varying increase in the number of glial cells involving the mediobasal portion of the temporal lobe. It is frequently accompanied by temporal lobe atrophy or hypoplasia. However, the majority of patients scanned for intractable temporal lobe epilepsy as a preoperative work-up do not show an MR abnormality, even when shown in many cases to have mesial temporal sclerosis pathologically. Unilateral temporal lobe atrophy is often difficult to assess, primarily because slight degrees of rotation of the head can give rise to considerable asymmetry of the images. Motion artifacts from CSF in the perimesencephalic cisterns may project over the mesial temporal lobes, particularly on T2-weighted images, when phase-encoding is from side to side. The cause of mesial temporal sclerosis is unknown; however, intrauterine hydrocephalus with entrapment of the posterior choroidal artery against the tentorial incisura leading to arterial compromise is mentioned frequently.

References

1. Schorner W, Meencke HJ, Felix R. Temporal lobe epilepsy: comparison of CT and MR imaging. *AJR* 1987;8:733–781.
2. Jack CR Jr, Gehring DG, Sharbrough FW, et al. Temporal lobe volume measurement in MR images: accuracy in left-right asymmetry in normal persons. *JCAT* 1988;12:21.
3. Triulzi F, Franceschi M, Fazio F, Del Maschio A. Non-refractory temporal lobe epilepsy: 1.5 T MR imaging. *Radiology* 1988;166:181.
4. Maertens PM, Machen BC, Williams JP et al. Magnetic resonance imaging of mesial temporal sclerosis: case reports. *J Comput Tomogr,* 1987;11:136.

Submitted by: Stephen J. Davis, M.D. and Louis M. Teresi, M.D., Huntington Medical Research Institutes, Pasadena, California; William G. Bradley, Jr., M.D., Ph.D., Senior Editor.

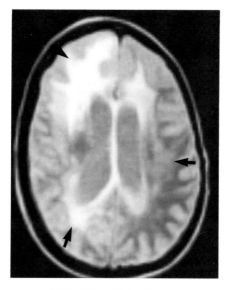

FIG. 92A. SE 2,000/60.

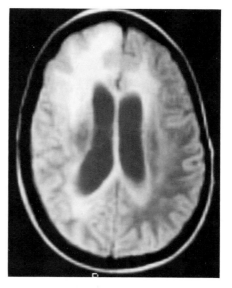

FIG. 92B. SE 2,000/30.

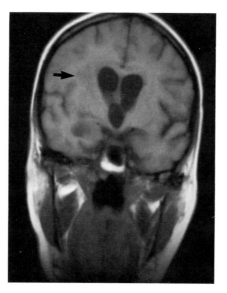

FIG. 92C. SE 500/30.

Clinical History

A 36-year-old female two years after whole brain irradiation.

Findings

Axial T2-W (SE 2,000/30 and 60) and coronal T1-W (SE 500/30) images are provided for review. On the T2-weighted axial images, diffuse high signal is noted in the white matter bilaterally, predominating in the right frontal lobe (92A, arrows). The coronal T1-weighted image shows that the white matter on the right (92C, arrow) is slightly hypointense relative to the white matter on the left. The right lateral ventricle is also slightly larger than the left.

Diagnosis

Radiation-induced demyelination.

Discussion

Radiation causes thickening and hyalinization of the arteriolar wall. Evidence suggesting that the associated demyelination results from the vascular changes included a long interval preceding the onset of symptoms, fibrinoid changes in arteriolar walls in the affected area, the severest changes in the white matter occurring in deep locations adjacent to the ventricle where blood supply is most tenuous, and high correlation between the severity of vascular change and the severity of demyelination. The MR appearance of radiation-induced demyelination is irregular and flame-shaped, extending to the more richly vascularized gray matter in severe cases, and affecting all white matter tracts. The corpus callosum is characteristically spared. The white matter in the radiation port is often the most severely affected when an asymmetric dose is applied. When the radiation dose is uniform, the forceps major may be more severely affected than the more anterior white matter tracts. This may reflect the fact that the penetrating arterioles posteriorly must traverse a longer course to penetrate the thicker fiber bundles in this area, whereas tracts of the corpus callosum are fed directly by short perforators from pial arteries from the anterior cerebral and posterior pericallosal arteries.

References

1. Curnes JT, Laster DW, Ball MR, et al. Magnetic resonance imaging of radiation injury to the brain. *AJNR* 1986;7:389–394.
2. Tsuruda JS, Kortman KE, Bradley WG, et al. Radiation effects on cerebral white matter: MR evaluation. *AJNR* 1987;8:431–437.

Submitted by: Louis M. Teresi, M.D., Stephen J. Davis, M.D., and Mark Ziemba, M.D., Huntington Medical Research Institutes, Pasadena, California; William G. Bradley, Jr., M.D., Ph.D., Senior Editor.

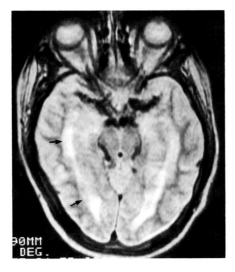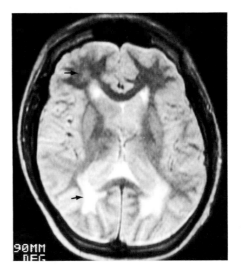

FIG. 93A. SE 2,000/84.   FIG. 93B. SE 2,000/84.

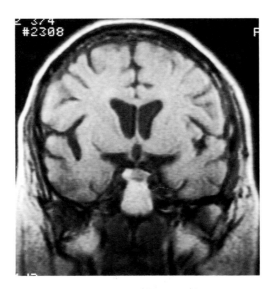

FIG. 93C. SE 667/28.

Clinical History

A 22-year-old male with a history of whole-brain radiation and methotrexate chemotherapy for leukemia, now complaining of lethargy.

Findings

Axial T2-W (SE 2,000/84) and coronal T1-W (SE 667/28) images are provided for review. The T2-weighted images show marked increased signal intensity in the white matter of the parietal and occipital lobes and moderate increased signal intensity in the frontal lobes (93A, 93B, arrows). Coronal T1-weighted images show no relative change in signal intensity of the white matter (93C). Diffuse cerebral atrophy is also noted.

Diagnosis

Diffuse necrotizing leukoencephalopathy (DNL).

Discussion

DNL is a syndrome that affects patients who have been treated with CNS radiation and chemotherapy, primarily intrathecal or intravenous methotrexate. Radiation therapy and chemotherapy are synergistic with respect to the CNS damage they elicit. Radiation disrupts the blood-brain barrier and increases the entry of chemotherapeutic drugs into the brain parenchyma thus potentiating their effects. Onset occurs shortly after completion of therapy. It is characterized clinically by a subacute course, the initial symptoms of which are confusion, ataxia, seizures, slurred speech, spasticity, dysphagia, and lethargy. Pathologic characteristics of this lesion include extensive areas of white matter demyelination and necrosis, astrocytosis, and a lack of inflammatory cellular response. MR findings in DNL are non-specific and include symmetric and asymmetric regions of high signal intensity in the white matter on T2-weighted images.

Reference

1. Ebner F, Ranner G, Slavc I, et al. MR findings in methotrexate-induced CNS abnormalities. *AJNR* 1988;10:959.

Submitted by: Louis M. Teresi, M.D., Stephen J. Davis, M.D., and Mark Ziemba, M.D., Huntington Medical Research Institutes, Pasadena, California; William G. Bradley, Jr., M.D., Ph.D., Senior Editor.

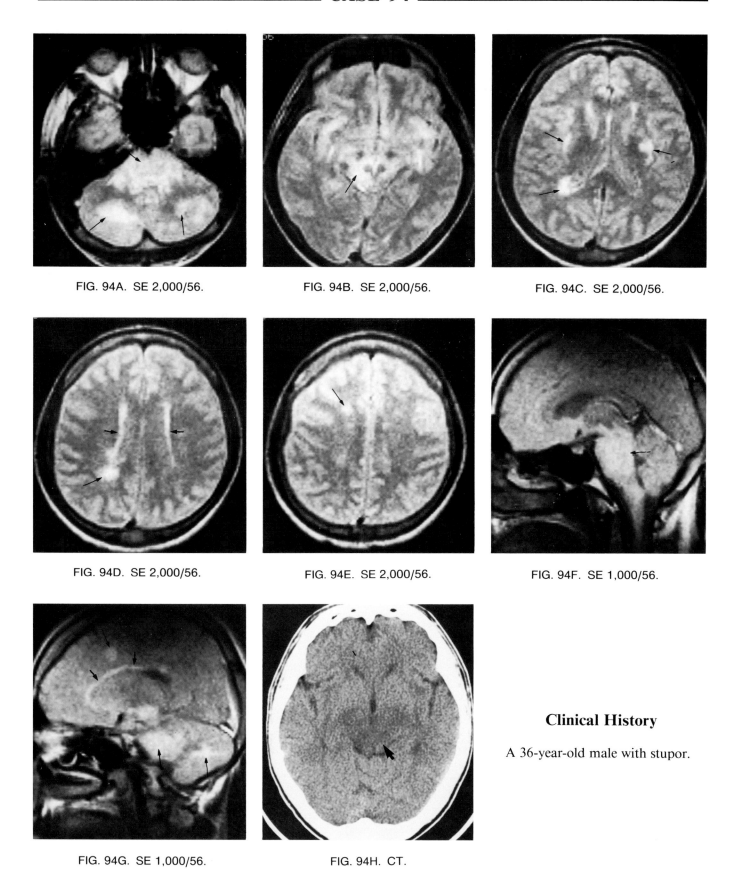

FIG. 94A. SE 2,000/56.

FIG. 94B. SE 2,000/56.

FIG. 94C. SE 2,000/56.

FIG. 94D. SE 2,000/56.

FIG. 94E. SE 2,000/56.

FIG. 94F. SE 1,000/56.

FIG. 94G. SE 1,000/56.

FIG. 94H. CT.

Clinical History

A 36-year-old male with stupor.

Findings

T2-weighted axial (SE 2,000/56), sagittal (SE 1,000/56) and non-contrast CT images are provided for review. T2-weighted images show multiple foci of increased signal intensity in the pons, cerebellar, and cerebral white matter (94A–94E, long arrows). The pons and midbrain are most prominently affected, being virtually replaced by high signal. High signal intensity is also noted in the ependyma of the lateral ventricles bilaterally (94D, short arrows). Sagittal (SE 1,000/56) images show to better advantage the cephalocaudal extent of the high signal abnormalities in the pons and midbrain (94F, arrow). Increased signal in the ependyma of the lateral ventricles (94G, short arrows) and in the cerebellar and cerebral white matter (94G, long arrows) persists on the SE 1,000/56 images. Non-contrast CT shows low density in the pons corresponding to the region of high signal intensity on the MR images (94H, arrow).

Diagnosis

Disseminated encephalitis, predominating in the brainstem; probable ventriculitis.

Discussion

Most acute viral encephalitides are relatively similar on MR and appear as scattered areas of high intensity on T2-weighted images, secondary to edema and necrosis. Paramagnetic contrast agents may make the early foci of encephalitis more conspicuous. Enhancement may be heterogeneous, gyriform, or leptomeningeal as subarachnoid extension of infection occurs. Postinfectious encephalomyelitis (acute disseminated encephalomyelitis) has a nonspecific appearance similar to the acute viral infections, especially measles, varicella, and rubella, or to vaccinations in the preceding weeks. The etiology is probably autoimmune with the development of delayed hypersensitivity to myelin basic protein or with the deposition of antigen-antibody complexes resulting in vasculitis. Pathologically, multiple perivenular zones of demyelination are associated with perivascular inflammation. On T2-weighted MR images, multiple areas of high-signal intensity in the white matter appear. Inflammatory cortical lesions may also be seen. All of these areas may be expected to enhance with contrast agents. In subacute sclerosing panencephalitis (SSPE), an atypical viral infection occurring years after the acute episode, the inflammatory changes may be so gradual that MR scans may show only atrophy. This is also noted to occur in Creutzfeldt-Jakob disease.

Long-term sequelae of the encephalitides include areas of demyelination and encephalomalacia, which are visible as regions of high intensity without mass effect on T2-weighted images. Small regions of demyelination contain increased water due to the loss of the hydrophobic myelin. MR is more sensitive than CT in its ability to detect these residual lesions.

Brain stem encephalitis is manifested by symptoms that include ataxia, hyporeflexia, ophthalmoplegia, and other cranial nerve palsies. In severe cases, respiratory compromise may ensue due to medullary involvement. While CT is usually unrevealing, MR may show high intensity in the brain stem consistent with encephalitis. The mass effect may be sufficient to locally expand the brain stem and compress the 4th ventricle and basal cisterns. The appearance can resemble a brain stem glioma. Specific pathogens vary. Brain stem encephalitis may follow nonspecific viral exanthems. In addition, although varicella-zoster virus can cause a diffuse meningoencephalites, in the Ramsey Hunt syndrome the latent virus in the facial nerve ganglia reactivates and spreads retrograde where it may involve the brain stem and cause a localized encephalitis. Rarely, herpes simplex virus can also spread in a similar retrograde fashion along the glossopharyngeal or vagus nerves and result in localized brain stem encephalitis.

References

1. Leetsma JG. Viral infections of the nervous system. In: Davis RL, Robertson DM, eds. *Textbook of neuropathology.* Baltimore: Williams and Wilkins, 1985.
2. Bradley WG, Bydder G. Demyelinating disease and infection. In: *MRI atlas of the brain.* London: Martin Dunitz, 1990;186.

Submitted by: Louis M. Teresi, M.D., Stephen J. Davis, M.D., and Mark Ziemba, M.D., Huntington Medical Research Institutes, Pasadena, California; William G. Bradley, Jr., M.D., Ph.D., Senior Editor.

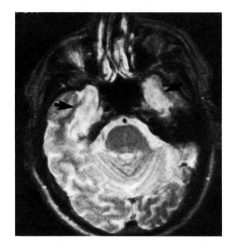
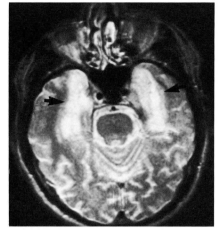

FIG. 95A. SE 2,500/70.

FIG. 95B. SE 2,500/70.

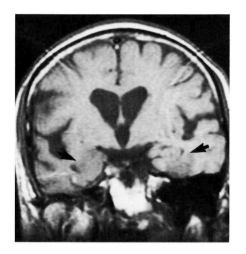

FIG. 95C. SE 600/20.

Clinical History

A 76-year-old man with a history of lethargy and confusion.

Findings

Axial T2-W (SE 2,500/70) and coronal T1-W (SE 600/20) images are provided for review. The T2-weighted images show diffuse increased signal intensity in the mesiotemporal lobes bilaterally (95A, 95B, arrows). Corresponding regions of decreased signal intensity are noted on the coronal T1-weighted images (95C, arrow).

Diagnosis

Herpes encephalitis.

Discussion

Herpes simplex has a predilection for the antero-inferior portions of the temporal lobe and the limbic system. Involvement may be unilateral or bilateral. The inferior surfaces of the frontal lobes are also occasionally involved. MRI findings are relatively specific, based on the location of involvement—uncus, hippocampal gyrus, parahippocampal gyrus, putamen, external capsule. MRI is much more sensitive than CT due to its ability to detect subtle increases in brain water, represented as high signal on T2-weighted images. Foci of hemorrhage may also be visible as punctate areas of high intensity on both T1- and T2-weighted images. This is of importance in herpes simplex encephalitis, as early institution of antiviral agents, such as acyclovir, has been demonstrated to be of great importance in limiting the sequelae of the disease.

Reference

1. Davidson HD, Steiner RE. MRI in infections of the central nervous system. *AJNR* 1985;6:499–504.

Submitted by: Louis M. Teresi, M.D., Stephen J. Davis, M.D., and Mark Ziemba, M.D., Huntington Medical Research Institutes, Pasadena, California; William G. Bradley, Jr., M.D., Ph.D., Senior Editor.

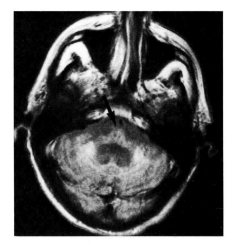

FIG. 96A. SE 2,000/30.

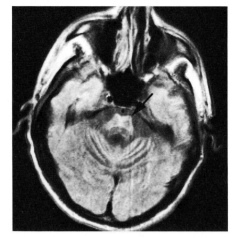

FIG. 96B. SE 2,000/30.

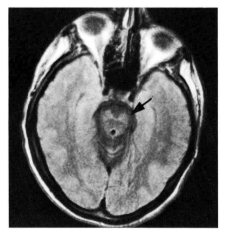

FIG. 96C. SE 2,000/30.

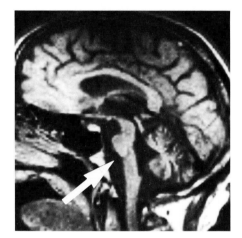

FIG. 96D. SE 500/40.

Clinical History

A 55-year-old male with ataxia and fine motor incoordination.

Findings

Axial T2-W (SE 2,000/30) and sagittal T1-W (SE 500/50) images are provided for review. Images show severe atrophy of the pons and cerebellum (96A–96D, arrows). The supratentorial structures show a normal mild degree of atrophy for age and no abnormal signal intensity.

Diagnosis

Olivopontocerebellar degeneration.

Discussion

Olivopontocerebellar atrophy, which may occur in a sporadic form (Dejerine and André Thomas Type) or in a familial form (Menzel Type), has its onset in middle life with progressive cerebellar ataxia, scanning speech, dysarthria, and cranial nerve involvement. There is neuronal depopulation and degeneration of the olivocerebellar and pontocerebellar fibers. Cerebellar atrophy follows and there is severe demyelination with gliosis of the central cerebellar white matter. The basal ganglia, especially the substantia nigra and dentate nuclei, are variably affected. MR findings are characteristic, showing atrophy of the pons and cerebellum.

Reference

1. Escouroulle R, Poirier J. *Manual of neuropathology.* Philadelphia: W. B. Saunders Company, 1978; 141–142.

Submitted by: Louis M. Teresi, M.D., Stephen J. Davis, M.D., and Mark Ziemba, M.D., Huntington Medical Research Institutes, Pasadena, California; William G. Bradley, Jr., M.D., Ph.D., Senior Editor.

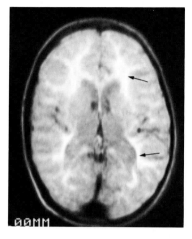

FIG. 97A. SE 1,984/84.

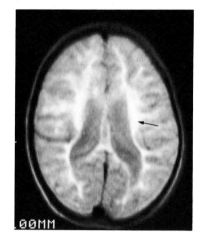

FIG. 97B. SE 1,984/84.

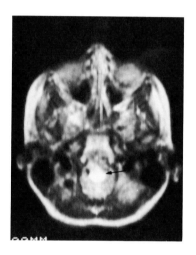

FIG. 97C. SE 1,984/84.

Clinical History

A 9-year-old female with nystagmus and poor head control.

Findings

Axial T2-W (SE 1,984/84) images are provided for review. The white matter has increased signal intensity diffusely (97A, 97B, arrows). Of particular note is the increased signal intensity of the brainstem (97C, arrow).

Diagnosis

Pelizaeus-Merzbacher disease.

Discussion

Pelizaeus-Merzbacher disease is a rare sex-linked recessive condition manifest in early infancy with a protracted clinical course. The disease is characterized by speech abnormalities, grimacing, ataxia, choreiform movements, spasticity, and mental deterioration. Pathologically, the disease consists of a dysmyelinating process in which small islands of normal myelin, often perivascular in distribution, are found to persist along the main nerve fiber pathways. Axons are well preserved, and there is striking contrast between the severity of the myelin changes and the paucity of macrophage reaction. Pathologically, there is sclerosis of the white matter of the cerebrum and cerebellum. There are subtle characteristic regions of loss of myelin throughout the brain.

References

1. Van der Knapp MS, Valk J. The reflection of histology in MR imaging of Pelizaeus-Merzbacher disease. *AJNR* 1989;10:99–105.
2. Escouroulle R, Poirier J. *Manual of neuropathology.* Philadelphia: W. B. Saunders Company, 1978;130–131.

Submitted by: Louis M. Teresi, M.D., Stephen J. Davis, M.D., and Mark Ziemba, M.D., Huntington Medical Research Institutes, Pasadena, California; William G. Bradley, Jr., M.D., Ph.D., Senior Editor.

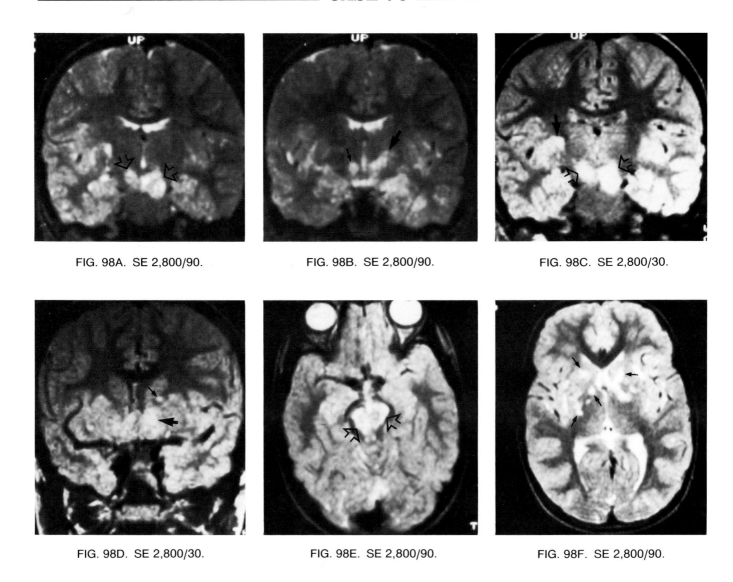

FIG. 98A. SE 2,800/90.

FIG. 98B. SE 2,800/90.

FIG. 98C. SE 2,800/30.

FIG. 98D. SE 2,800/30.

FIG. 98E. SE 2,800/90.

FIG. 98F. SE 2,800/90.

Clinical History

An 8-year-old female with history of diplopia, bilateral weakness, and lethargy.

Findings

Axial T2-W (SE 2,800/90) and coronal T2-W (SE 2,800/30 and 90) images are provided for review. T2-weighted images (98A–98F) show large regions of increased signal intensity in the upper pons (open arrows) and innumerable smaller high signal regions scattered throughout the basal ganglia and internal capsules bilaterally (solid arrows).

Diagnosis

Leigh's disease.

Discussion

Leigh's disease, or subacute necrotizing encephalopathy, is seen most often in early childhood, but variants with late onset have been described. The condition is characterized by the presence of symmetrical spongy necrotizing lesions that affect the cortex and sometimes the hemispheric white matter. Involvement of the basal ganglia, tegmentum of the brainstem, corpora quadrigemina, and inferior olivae is characteristic. There is relative sparing of the neurons, the presence of gliosis, and especially the endothelial proliferation. There is thought to be a metabolic disorder responsible for the lesions, perhaps a disturbance of the Kreb's cycle. This is poorly understood, however.

MR demonstrates multiple foci of increased signal intensity involving both gray and white matter. In addition to the abnormalities of the lentiform nuclei frequently documented by CT, lesions are shown in the brainstem and cortical gray matter.

References

1. Davis PC, Hoffman JC, Braun IF. MR imaging of Leigh's disease. *AJNR* 1987;8:71–77.
2. Escouroulle R, Poirier J. *Manual of neuropathology.* Philadelphia: W. B. Saunders Company, 1978; 141–142.

Submitted by: Louis M. Teresi, M.D., Stephen J. Davis, M.D., and Mark Ziemba, M.D., Huntington Medical Research Institutes, Pasadena, California; William G. Bradley, Jr., M.D., Ph.D., Senior Editor.

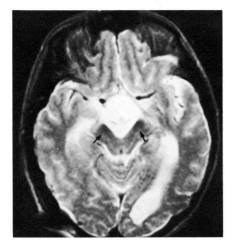

FIG. 99A. SE 3,000/90.

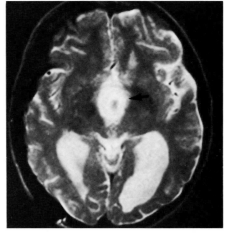

FIG. 99B. SE 3,000/90.

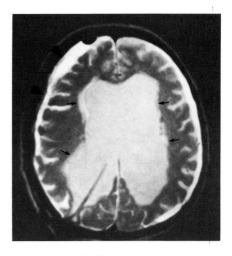

FIG. 99C. SE 3,000/90.

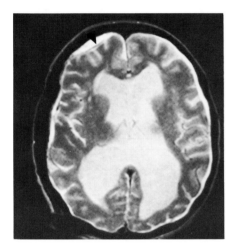

FIG. 99D. SE 3,000/90.

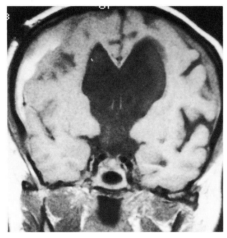

FIG. 99E. SE 800/20.

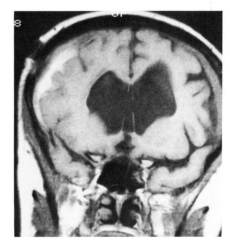

FIG. 99F. SE 800/20.

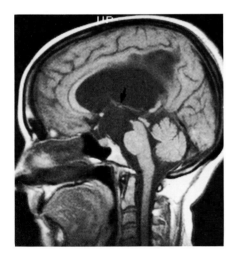

FIG. 99G. SE 500/17.

Clinical History

A 41-year-old female with a history of repeated shunt revision for obstructive hydrocephalus. Can you see what is causing the obstruction?

Findings

Axial T2-W (SE 3,000/90), sagittal T1-W (SE 500/17), and coronal T1-W (SE 800/20) images are provided for review. Marked enlargement is noted of the lateral and 3rd ventricles. The T2-weighted axial images (99C, arrows) show a thin rim of hyperintensity around the lateral ventricles. Lower axial images show that the 3rd ventricle has an expanded appearance (99B, arrow), and there is splaying of the cerebral peduncles (99A, arrows). The midline sagittal image provides a better perspective of the enlarged 3rd ventricle and also shows upward displacement of the fornix (99G, arrow). The size of the 4th ventricle is normal, as is size of the aqueduct.

Bilateral subdural fluid collections are seen on the axial T2-weighted (99C) and coronal T1-weighted (99E, 99F) images. The collection on the left is isointense on the T1-weighted images and hyperintense on the T2-weighted images. The collection on the right has two components: (1) an outer area that is isointense on the T1-weighted images and hyperintense on the T2-weighted images and (2) an inner area that is hyperintense on both T1- and T2-weighted images. A thickened subdural membrane is also seen on the T2-weighted axial images (99C, 99D, arrowheads).

Diagnosis

Suprasellar arachnoid cyst; left chronic subdural hematoma; right subacute to chronic subdural hematoma.

Discussion

Arachnoid cysts account for about 1% of all intracranial mass lesions, but fewer than 15% are located in the suprasellar region. The membrane of Liliequist has been suggested to play a role in the development of suprasellar arachnoid cysts. This normally perforated, veil-like membrane incompletely separates the interpeduncular and the chiasmatic parts of the suprasellar cistern, stretching between its attachment points at the dorsum sella, oculomotor nerves, hypothalamus, and ventral midbrain. Theoretically, imperforation of this membrane, secondary to congenital maldevelopment or acquired adhesive arachnoiditis, produces obstruction of cerebrospinal flow from the infratentorial to the supratentorial subarachnoid spaces. The continued egress of CSF from the 4th ventricle causes upward expansion of the membrane in the suprasellar cistern, resulting in formation of a diverticulum that communicates with the pontine cistern. Further enlargement results in progressive invagination of the diverticulum through the hypothalamus into the 3rd ventricle and even through the foramina of Monro into the lateral ventricles. Most patients develop symptoms during infancy, secondary to obstructive hydrocephalus; however, other patients may not present until the second or third decade.

Prior to MR, CT with intrathecal contrast administration was the conventional method of diagnosing suprasellar arachnoid cysts. Direct sagittal scanning with MR can assist with the diagnosis. Superior extension of the cyst from the suprasellar cistern into the anterior aspect of the 3rd ventricle commonly results in superior displacement and lateral separation of the anterior columns of the fornix. On axial images, the 3rd ventricle is enlarged and there is characteristic splaying of the cerebral peduncles.

The differentiation of suprasellar arachnoid cyst from suprasellar cystic neoplasms is usually possible by the homogeneous appearance of the suprasellar arachnoid cyst, with signal intensity similar to CSF, visualization of the paper-thin wall of the cysts where they are adjacent to the lateral or 3rd ventricles, and the lack of calcification and fat. Although a suprasellar arachnoid cyst may bear resemblance to a dilated 3rd ventricle associated with distal obstruction, they can be differentiated on the basis of the shape and contour of the apparent 3rd ventricle, characteristic parasellar mass effect and displacement of adjacent structures, and distinctive basal cisternal expansion.

Reference

1. Gentry LR, Smoker WR, Turski PA. Suprasellar arachnoid cysts: CT recognition. *AJNR* 1986;7:79–86.

Submitted by: Louis M. Teresi, M.D., Stephen J. Davis, M.D., and Mark Ziemba, M.D., Huntington Medical Research Institutes, Pasadena, California; William G. Bradley, Jr., M.D., Ph.D., Senior Editor.

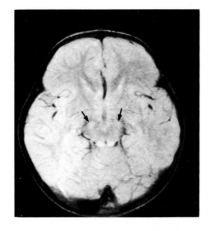

FIG. 100A. SE 2,000/60.

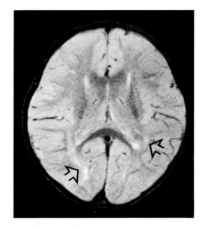

FIG. 100B. SE 2,000/60.

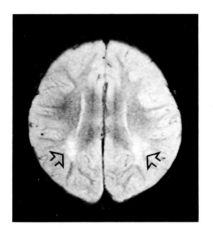

FIG. 100C. SE 2,000/60.

Clinical History

An 18-month-old with a history of seizures, behavioral disturbances, and left hemiparesis.

Findings

Axial T2-W (SE 2,000/60) images are provided for review. The axial SE 2,000/60 images show increased signal intensity in the white matter of the occipital lobes (100B, 100C, arrows). Increased signal intensity is also noted in the cerebral peduncles bilaterally (100A, arrows).

Diagnosis

Adrenoleukodystrophy.

Discussion

Adrenoleukodystrophy is a hereditary disorder that involves the adrenal cortex and white matter of the CNS. Clinical symptoms include behavioral disturbances, mental deterioration, motor dysfunction, dysphagia, decreased vision, and seizures. The disease leads to death. Features of adrenal insufficiency may precede, concur, or follow neurologic symptoms. The basic metabolic defect is an impaired capacity to degrade very-long-chain fatty acids, which is caused by paroxysmal defect in beta-oxidation. The increasing accumulation of fatty acids with very long chains probably decreases the stability of the myelin membrane, finally leading to demyelination. MR images reflect demyelination as hyperintensity on T2-weighted images. Areas characteristically involved in adrenoleukodystrophy include the occipital white matter with relative sparing of the subcortical U-fibers, the splenium of the corpus callosum, medial and lateral geniculate bodies, cerebellar white matter, and the corticospinal tracts.

Reference

1. Van der Knapp MS, Valk J. MR of adrenoleukodystrophy: histopathologic correlations. *AJNR* 1989;10:12.

Submitted by: Louis M. Teresi, M.D., Stephen J. Davis, M.D., and Mark Ziemba, M.D., Huntington Medical Research Institutes, Pasadena, California; William G. Bradley, Jr., M.D., Ph.D., Senior Editor.

NOTE: An *f* following a page number indicates an illustration.